Copyright @2019 by Zondra Wilson & Keith Bossier

All scripture quotations, unless otherwise noted, are taken from the Holy Bible; New International Version (North American Edition). Copyright 1973, 1978, 1984 by International Bible Society. Used by permission of Zondervan. All rights reserved.

The "N.I.V." and "New International Version" trademarks are registered in the United States Patent and Trademark Office by International Bible Society.

Requests for information should be addressed to:
Zondra Wilson
12700 Inglewood Blvd.
#1623
Hawthorne, CA 90251
zondraSwilson@yahoo.com

Printed in the United States of America

Table of Contents

"IN THE BEGINNING WAS THE WORD, AND THE WORD WAS WITH GOD, AND THE WORD WAS GOD" JOHN 1:1(NIV)

This is one of my favorite scriptures. It reminds me of how things often start - with a Word! My dreams, visions and overall way of life all started with a Word from God! I can remember as a child growing up in Cleveland trying to figure out what I wanted to do with my life. I eventually chose the path of becoming a news anchor/reporter. Although I loved my career, deep down inside, I knew something was missing. I always enjoyed helping people and found the perfect opportunity when Michigan was declared the fattest state in America. I wanted to do something about it. So, I got certified through the American Council on Exercise (ACE) as a personal trainer. My goal was to implement small steps for parishioners to obtain better health. It worked! I felt so fulfilled. This started me on my health and wellness journey in helping people with their fitness goals.

I then felt a nudge from the Holy Spirit to move to Los Angeles and pursue acting. But the one thing that was always there "in the beginning" was fitness. Although my diet wasn't the healthiest, I always worked out. Initially, I did it just to stay slim. Then one day, "the word" from my doctor during a routine office visit changed my life. "Ms. Wilson, you are pre-diabetic." I was stunned. I asked her, "What exactly does that mean?" I was confused because I was slim and looked a picture of health on the outside. But what the doctor explained to me is that my inside told a different story. The doctor went on to say that eventually my inside was going to start showing on the outside. It was my wakeup call to not only concentrate on my "outer" body but my "inner" body as well.

So, what exactly is Pre-diabetes? Pre-diabetes is a warning that you're on the path to diabetes. My doctor told me that it wasn't too late for me to turn things around. If you have it (like 86 million other Americans), your blood sugar (glucose) level is higher than it should be, but not in the diabetes range. People used to call it "borderline" diabetes. Pre-diabetes makes you more likely to get heart disease or have a stroke. But you can take action to lower those risks through diet and exercise. Unfortunately, there are usually no symptoms. Only a doctor can diagnose you for sure. Lifestyle changes can help many people with pre-diabetes delay or prevent it from becoming diabetes.

But like many others, I underestimated my sugar intake. I would chew gum just to suck the sweet out, spit it out and pop another piece into my mouth. I would chew packs of this stuff everyday. After meeting with a nutritionist, I made a conscious effort to change my eating habits because I refused to take medication. I wanted to develop a healthier lifestyle the way God intended. I started chewing sugar-free gum and eliminated the endless snacking on sweets between meals. I adopted a healthy diet rich in fruits, vegetables and whole grains. Not only did my LDL cholesterol level drop, but stubborn fat and inches just melted away.

So, what is LDL cholesterol? It's the type that puts your heart at risk and is sometimes called the "bad" cholesterol. It collects in the walls of your blood vessels, where it can cause blockages. Higher levels of LDL can raise your chances of a heart attack. That's because of a sudden blood clot that forms there.

Get a simple blood test from your doctor to check your LDL levels. If it's high, healthy foods and medicine can help you get them down. According to some doctors, LDL cholesterol levels should be less than 100 mg/dl. Levels of 100 to 129 mg/dl are acceptable for people with no health issues but may be of more concern for those with heart disease or heart disease risk factors. A reading of 130 to 159 mg/dl is borderline high and 160 to 189 mg/dl is high. Always consult your doctor about your individual cholesterol levels for any diagnosis.

Also, as we age (especially 40 and up), our bodies require fewer calories. Why? Metabolism! Metabolism is your body's ability to break down nutrients and convert them into energy. The bottom line is that I could no longer eat the same amount of food and exercise the same way to achieve my ideal body as I did in my 20's.

So, I went into fervent prayer asking God for strength to help me with this next chapter in my life. I wanted to carry out God's work with a strong and healthy mind and body. During prayer, I heard the Spirit tell me to put together a fitness video and write a book for people 40 and over. But, there was a problem. I had left the fitness industry because I wanted to concentrate on acting. So, here we go again. God messing in my life. LOL!

But I'm an Actress!

"Have I not commanded you? Be strong and courageous. Do not be afraid; do not be discouraged, for the LORD your God will be with you wherever you go." **Joshua 1:9 (NIV)**

In my mind, I would always say, "Lord if you want me to start on this venture, then provide the vision and money." I remember God saying, *"Trust in the Lord with all your heart and lean not unto your own understanding. In all your ways, acknowledge him and he will direct your path".* **Proverbs 3:5-6 (NIV)** God quickly granted me peace.

Looking back, I know that the whole situation was in God's hand. He was preparing me to move to another level in my life. Although it wasn't what I had in mind, it was the best possible plan for my future.

The Lesson of Faith!

Trust! I learned to **trust**. I learned to **trust** what I hear from God. That has been an issue with me because I was living my life the way I saw fit, instead of according to the instruction of the Holy Spirit. I have learned to **trust** God with everything, from how I exercise, to what I eat, to the clothes that I wear.

My Abundant Living!

Not only did God guide me in starting ***"Faithful, Forty & Fabulously Fit"***, He also blessed me with the idea of starting Blu Skin Care, LLC. Blu Skin Care manufactures and produces USDA certified organic skin care products (www.bluskincare.info). I thought, "I'm an actress. It makes more sense for me to produce movies and films." The seasoned Saints would say - "Do you want to make God laugh? Tell Him your plans for your life." They *ain't neva* lied! LOL!

What it's taught me in my life is to listen to Him, no matter how crazy the message may sound. No matter what my circumstances look like, I need to **trust** what He's telling me to do. I had to SURRENDER my will to His. I have to **trust** that He will guide me all the way. - Zondra

How To Apply!

The first thing is to allow The Holy Spirit to train you to hear from Him in every area of your life. Daily, pray and ask for discernment regarding your fitness goals, business operations and the studying/interpretation of scripture.

You also have to start off with *worship*. *Worship Him* to get your body and mind in a place where you can hear Him. This is so important to know for certain if it's your flesh, the enemy or God speaking to you. Remember, you can *worship* God anywhere and at any time. I love to turn on Pandora and listen to gospel music during my *worship* experiences. However, some may choose to *worship* through meditation or the reading of scripture. *Worship* the way God leads you. It's all about pleasing Him.

Steps to Getting Started

Planning and preparation are important when you're getting started with exercise, but to be successful, you also need momentum—and the more you can create, the easier it is to stay motivated. The best way to build and maintain momentum is with action. While it's great to ponder your weight loss goals, think about motivation and work on your commitment to exercise. There's something to be said for just doing it—before too much contemplation drains your energy.

Step 1: Record Your Measurements

This isn't a must, but tracking your progress has many benefits, especially if your goal is to lose weight. In addition to keeping you accountable to yourself and committed to achieving your goals, it makes it more likely you'll reach—and even surpass—them.

Weighing yourself and keeping an exercise journal are two ways to track your progress, but taking your measurements (chest, arms, waist, hips) will give you a little more information. For example, you may be losing inches even if the scale number doesn't go down. In that case, monitoring your measurements every few weeks can reassure you that you are inching closer to your ideal size.

Step 2: Get Your Doctor's Clearance

If you have any injuries, illnesses or conditions, or are on any medications, talk to your doctor to make sure it's okay to exercise. Some medications may affect your heart rate and it's important to know if you have to adjust your workouts.

Step 3: Prepare to Work Out

When it comes to slimming down and toning up, there are two key types of workouts: cardio, which burns calories by raising your heart rate, and strength training, which builds the lean muscle that boosts metabolism, the rate at which you burn calories. Together, this pairing can produce powerful weight-loss results.

Cardio workouts are designed to be done on any cardio machine (treadmill, elliptical, bike, or rowing machine). However, you are free to choose other cardio activities (for instance, running, cycling, fitness videos, or group fitness classes). These are all good cardio workouts.

For the strength workouts, you'll need some equipment:

- *Various weighted dumbbells.* Some exercises require heavier weights, while others will need lighter weights or none at all. Try to have a range of dumbbells: a light set (3 to 5 pounds for women, 5 to 8 pounds for men), a medium set (5 to 10 pounds for women, 10 to 15 pounds for men), and a heavy set (10 to 20 pounds for women, 15 to 30 pounds for men).

- *An exercise ball.* These giant balls are one of the best tools to strengthen the abs and back and increase stability. They come in different sizes to accommodate your height. When you sit on one, there should be a 90-degree angle at your hip and knee joints.

- *An exercise mat.* Yoga mats are thinner and have more gripping ability to hold poses. Thicker mats are best for Pilates and abdominal exercises because they cushion the spine while you're lying on your back.

It will also help to know the basics of weight training, including two key terms: reps and sets.

Rep, or repetition, is a single instance of an exercise—a dumbbell bicep curl, for instance.

A set is the number of repetitions performed sequentially.

For example, you can say, "I did 3 sets of 15 reps of bicep curls."

Also important to know is how to determine how much weight you should use (if any). Start with a light set of dumbbells/weights and perform a set. Continue adding weight until you can do the desired number of reps with good form, which includes moving slowly enough that you're using muscle—and not momentum—to lift the weight. The last rep should be difficult, but not impossible, and you should be able to keep good form while doing it.

HEALTHY EATING!

Find your healthy eating style. Everything you eat and drink over time matters and can help you be healthier now and in the future.

- Focus on whole fruits.
- Vary your veggies.
- Move to low-fat or fat-free milk or yogurt.
- Make half your grains whole grains.
- Vary your protein routine.
- Drink and eat beverages and food with less sodium, saturated fat and added sugars.
- Start with small changes that you can enjoy, like having an extra piece of fruit today.
- Add fruits & vegetables to your diet.
- Add grains to your diet.
- Add dairy proteins to your diet.
- Focus on whole fruits and select 100% fruit juice when choosing juices. (Buy fruits that are dried, frozen or fresh so that you can always have a supply on hand.)
- Eat a variety of vegetables and add them to mixed dishes like casseroles, sandwiches and wraps.
- Regarding your veggies; fresh, frozen and canned count too. Look for "reduced sodium" or "no-salt-

added" on the label.

•Choose whole-grain versions of common foods such as bread, pasta and tortillas.

Not sure if it's whole grain? Check the ingredients list for the words "whole" or "whole grain".

DAILY FOOD GROUP TARGETS – BASED ON A 2,000 CALORIE PLAN

1 cup counts as:
•2 cups raw spinach
•1 large bell pepper
•1 cup baby carrots
•1 cup green peas
•1 cup mushrooms
•1 large banana
•2 cup mandarin oranges
•1/2 cup raisins
•1 cup 100% grapefruit juice

1 ounce counts as:
- 1 slice of bread
- 1/2 cup cooked oatmeal
- 1 small tortilla
- 1/2 cup cooked brown rice
- 1/2 cup cooked grits

Choose low-fat (1%) or fat-free (skim) dairy. Get the same amount of calcium and other nutrients as whole milk, but with less saturated fat and calories.

Lactose intolerant? Try lactose-free milk or a fortified soy beverage.

1 cup counts as:
- 1 cup milk
- 1 cup yogurt
- 2 ounces processed cheese (you want to limit all processed foods)

Eat a variety of protein foods such as beans, soy, seafood, lean meats, poultry and unsalted nuts and seeds.
Select seafood twice a week. Choose lean cuts of meat and ground beef that is at least 93% lean.

1 ounce counts as:

- 1 ounce tuna fish
- 1/4 cooked beans
- 1 tbsp peanut butter
- 1 egg

Water

Drink water instead of sugary drinks.

Regular soda, energy or sports drinks and other sweet drinks usually contain a lot of added sugar which provides more calories than needed.

WHAT SHOULD YOU EAT ON A 1200 AND 1500 CALORIE DIET?

Use These Servings for a Balanced Reduced Calorie Weight Loss Diet

The Pyramid Diet

This is the diet developed by the USDA to satisfy the nutritional requirements of most Americans.

0-3 servings (use sparingly) fats, oils, sweets

2-3 servings (6 - 9 ounces) meat/protein

2-3 servings dairy

2-4 servings fruit
3-5 servings vegetables
6-11 servings bread/starch

In order to lose weight, you must take in fewer calories than you burn off each day. According to the USDA pamphlet, a sedentary woman and older people may only expend 1600 calories per day, while active men and very active women may burn 2800 calories per day - twice as much.

If your goal is to lose weight and you do not see changes just with increased physical activity, then reducing portions and servings may help. Be sure to use the pyramid as a guide.

1200 Calorie Diet

6 oz. lean meat/protein
5 servings bread/starch
3 servings fruit
4 or more servings vegetables
2 servings dairy (low fat preferred)
3 servings fat

1500 Calorie Diet

6 oz. lean meat/protein

6 servings bread/starch

4 servings fruit

5 or more servings vegetables

2 servings dairy (low fat preferred)

3 servings fat

What is a Serving?

How much is a serving? Follow these guidelines.

Bread, Cereal, Rice, and Pasta

1 slice of bread or tortilla (1 oz)

1/2 bagel or 1/2 english muffin or 1/2 pita (1 oz)

1 oz of ready to-eat cereal

1/2 cup of cooked cereal, rice, or pasta

Vegetables

1 cup of raw leafy vegetables

1/2 cup of other vegetables, cooked or chopped raw

1/2 cup of vegetable juice

(Some diets put raw leafy vegetables into a "free use" category - eat as much as you want of leaf lettuce, celery, radishes)

Fruit

1 medium apple, banana, orange

1 cup berries, cubed melon

1/2 cup of chopped, cooked, or canned fruit (be sure its low sodium)

1/2 cup of fruit juice

Milk, Yogurt, and Cheese

1 cup milk

1 cup yogurt

3/4 cup plain yogurt

1/4 cup cottage cheese or ricotta

1 oz cheese

Meat, Poultry, Fish, Dry Beans, Eggs, and Nuts

2-3 oz of cooked lean meat, poultry, or fish (3 oz. is about the size of a deck of cards)
1 - 1 1/2 cup of cooked beans
4-6 tablespoons of peanut butter or 1 cup of nuts
2-3 eggs

Fats

1 teaspoon oil, butter, margarine, mayonnaise
1 tablespoon salad dressing, cream cheese

Based on National Institutes of Health (1998) and American Diabetic Association Exchange List

SUPERFOODS

Processed foods fuel weight gain. Superfoods support weight loss!

Hunting for healthy options at the grocery store can sometimes feel like searching for a needle in a haystack. With unhealthy, processed foods lurking around every corner, it's no wonder that our country is facing an obesity epidemic.

Thankfully, nutritious food is available, if you know what to look for. Let us help you to navigate grocery store aisles with ease. Keep our "Ultimate Shopping List" of 50 superfoods handy, and you'll feel good about the nutritious items filling your cart the next time you shop. When you're armed with a great superfoods list, you can't go wrong in the store. Here are some other superfoods you can add to your grocery list.

1. Almonds
Few superfoods deserve a spot on this list as much as almonds.

2. Apples

"An apple a day keeps the doctor away".

3. Apricots

These orange-colored little fruits offer some great health benefits and are easy to snack on when you're on-the-go.

4. Artichokes

As long as you avoid drenching these fabulous green globes in mayo or butter, artichokes may actually help to lower your cholesterol.

5. Asparagus

This green stalky vegetable is fabulous at assisting the body in the removal of waste products. It tastes great when steamed, too!

6. Avocados

Avocados are pretty tough not to love. Not only do they pack quite a nutritional punch, they're incredibly satisfying, too!

7. Bananas

With their versatility and delicious taste, bananas may be one of the most pleasant ways to enhance your health.

8. Beans and Lentils
Beans and lentils provide a ton of fiber, protein, and a host of other health benefits.

9. Beets
You either love em' or hate em'. LOL!

10. Bell Peppers
Whether they're red, yellow, orange or green, bell peppers pack quite a nutritional punch. Bake them, broil them, steam them or eat them raw. Any way you slice them, bell peppers taste great!

11. Berries
For a fruit so small, berries are a true nutritional powerhouse!

12. Broccoli
When Mom told you to eat your broccoli, she knew what she was talking about!

13. Brussels Sprouts
When prepared correctly, brussel sprouts are one of the tastiest veggies around. They're great for your health, too!

14. Cabbage

If you love cabbage, feel free to brag to those who don't about all of the health benefits cabbage offers you.

15. Cantaloupe

This deliciously sweet melon is the perfect addition to a summer salad, and it can improve your health, too!

16. Carrots

Every kid knows that carrots are great for eyesight, but your vision isn't the only thing impacted by adding carrots.

17. Cauliflower

This cruciferous white veggie is packed with vitamin C and manganese and is excellent for your health.

18. Cherries

Cherries are one of those nutritional superfoods that you should devour while you have the chance. When cherry season arrives, you can feel good about what you're doing to preserve your brain and heart health. Cherries may be credited with slowing down the aging process and even with ending insomnia!

19. Chia Seeds

These tiny seeds are rich in omega-3 fatty acids and provide protein, healthy fats and fiber. Try adding two tablespoons to your favorite smoothie recipe.

20. Coconut

This tasty fruit is one of the most versatile superfoods out there.

21. Dark Chocolate

If you need a good excuse to eat your chocolate, look no further. Dark chocolate (not milk chocolate) may be great for cardiovascular health, premature aging and cancer. And guess what? Dark chocolate is low on the glycemic index!

22. Eggs

Full of protein and extremely versatile, eggs are rich in nutrients. They can tackle a number of health problems and encourage weight loss.

23. Fish

It's important to monitor which fish adds nutritional value without any health risks. If you find the good stuff, you'll reap amazing benefits. Fish may protect your heart, fight cancer, and strengthen your immune system.

24. Flax Seeds

This little seed is a nutritional powerhouse. It may help your digestion, strengthen your immune system and help with diabetes. The only seeds more powerful than flax are Chia seeds. But that doesn't mean you should forgo flax. It's far more readily available than Chia seeds are and it is often more cost-effective for those on a budget.

25. Garlic

Most folks these days know the benefits of eating garlic. Garlic may lower cholesterol, help with high blood pressure, fight against cancer and even kill certain bacteria.

26. Grapes

This fruit is fabulously portable, so there's no excuse not to include grapes in your healthy eating plan. They may strengthen your eyes, help with circulation and may even fight cancer and kidney stones.

27. Hot Peppers

Heat up your meals by adding hot peppers to your plate. They promise better digestion, an improved immune system and better blood circulation and digestion. There is even a rumor that hot peppers aid in weight loss by increasing your metabolism.

28. Kale

This superfood has powerful antioxidant qualities. Kale contains high amounts of phyto chemicals that may help in preventing macular degeneration and cataracts. Kale may also help to combat many types of cancer, including breast cancer. Include this antioxidant powerhouse in your morning smoothie.

29. Kiwi

Kiwi is different from many other fruits because it contains a number of beneficial substances instead of just one or two. Kiwis are full of antioxidants and make you feel as if you're on a tropical vacation with every bite.

30. Lemons and Limes

These sour fruits are amazing at so many things. They may fight everything from cancer to the common cold. Never miss a chance to include these in your eating plan.

31. Low-Fat Yogurt and Kefir

Choose plain, non-fat Greek yogurt to pack protein on top of the numerous benefits including increased bone strength, lowered cholesterol, a stronger immune system and better digestion. It may also be great for ulcers.

32. Mangoes

This tropical delight may help strengthen your memory as well as your digestion. It may also fight cancer and Alzheimer's disease.

33. Mushrooms

The lowly mushroom deserves to stand on a pedestal because of its medicinal uses. It may help control blood pressure and lower your cholesterol. And yes, like many other foods on this list, mushrooms may fight cancer too!

34. Oats

Oats are well-known for their potential cholesterol-lowering abilities. But did you know they may also improve the condition of your skin and help fight diabetes?

35. Olive Oil

Olive oil can (and should) be a part of many of your recipes. It may strengthen the heart, fight diabetes and cancer and can help with weight loss. For those with dry skin, it's an excellent way to cleanse your skin. Just put a little oil on a cotton ball and wipe clean.

36. Oranges

We all know that a nice glass of OJ goes well with just about any breakfast. But did you know that oranges may strengthen your immune system, fight cancer and strengthen your heart?

37. Papaya

Papaya is a nutritional powerhouse. This yellow/orange fruit provides a number of health benefits and will leave your skin looking fabulous too!

38. Peaches

These summertime treats are great for digestion and constipation.

39. Pineapple

Never miss a chance to eat pineapple! Not only is it absolutely delicious on a hot summer day, it may also strengthen your digestion, your bones, and can aid with weight loss.

40. Pumpkin

Some folks see pumpkins as something to carve once a year. But the truth is, your friendly jack-o'-lantern also provides tons of fiber and may control blood pressure and normalize heart function.

41. Pomegranates

These amazing fruits may have up to seven times the amount of antioxidants of green tea! Impressed? They may also fight cancer, reduce blood pressure and lower bad cholesterol.

42. Quinoa

This "super grain" is high in fiber, filled with protein and offers a pleasant nutty flavor. It cooks up like rice and is naturally gluten-free. If you haven't tried it already, it's easy to prepare and surprisingly satisfying!

43. Spinach

Popeye had the right idea. You have to eat your spinach to grow strong! Why? Spinach may help fight cancer, improve your cardiovascular health and improve brain function!

44. Spirulina

Don't let the idea of eating algae prevent you from enjoying all the benefits that spirulina has to offer. It is loaded with essential vitamins and nutrients. Toss it into a smoothie or add it to your favorite recipe and you won't even know it's there. (But your body will!)

45. Sprouts

Feasting on sprouts is a deliciously inexpensive way to reach total body nourishment. You'll be amazed at how many essential nutrients are packed into these tasty baby plants.

46. Sweet Potatoes

Healthy eaters know that sweet potatoes are a fantastic carb to include in your healthy eating plan! Why? Because they protect your vision, encourage a good mood, fight cancer and keep your bones strong.

47. Swiss Chard

If you've never heard of swiss chard before, you're missing out. This leafy vegetable is related to spinach and beets and packs quite a nutritional punch.

48. Tomatoes

Tomatoes may be big-time cancer fighters! They also help battle high cholesterol.

49. Walnuts

Easy to pack and snack on while out and about, nuts are loaded with healthy fats and offer a huge array of health benefits. Walnuts may be great for lowering cholesterol, fighting cancer and improving your memory.

50. Wild Caught Salmon

Wild caught salmon provides oodles of omega-3 essential fatty acids, a crucial bit of nutrition. But, that's not all. Salmon also provides many other vitamins like B3 and B12, which contribute to a healthy metabolism.

· These are just a few superfoods. Be sure to research which superfoods are best for your dietary needs.

83 HEALTHY RECIPE SUBSTITUTIONS

"Baking Hacks"

1. Black beans for flour

Swapping out flour for a can of black beans (drained and rinsed, of course) in brownies is a great way to cut out the gluten and fit in an extra dose of protein, Plus, they taste great. When baking, swap out 1 cup flour for 1 cup black bean puree (about a 15 oz can).

2. Whole wheat flour for white flour

In virtually any baked good, replacing white flour with whole wheat can add a whole new dimension of nutrients, flavor and texture. Because whole wheat includes the outer shell of the grain, it also provides an extra punch of fiber, which aids in digestion and can even lower the risk of diabetes and heart disease. For every cup of white flour, substitute 7/8 cup of whole-wheat.

3. Unsweetened applesauce for sugar

Using applesauce in place of sugar can give the necessary sweetness without the extra calories and sugar. While one cup of unsweetened applesauce contains only about 100 calories, a cup of sugar can pack in more than 770 calories! This swap is perfect for oatmeal raisin cookies. Pro tip: You can sub sugar for apple sauce in a 1:1 ratio, but for every cup of applesauce you use, reduce the amount of liquid in the recipe by 1/4 cup.

4. Unsweetened applesauce for oil or butter

Don't knock this one till you've tried it. The applesauce gives the right consistency and a hint of sweetness without all the fat of oil or butter. This works well in any sweet bread, like banana or zucchini, or in muffins – and even with pre-boxed mixes! On your first try, only try swapping out half the fat (so a recipe using 1 cup of oil would use 1/2 cup oil and 1/2 cup applesauce). If you can't tell the difference with that swap, try swapping a bit more of the fat next time around.

5. Almond flour for wheat flour

This gluten-free switch gives any baked good a dose of protein, omega-3s and a delicious nutty flavor. A word of advice: almond flour is much heavier than other baking flours, so when subbing go 1/4 cup at a time (so 1 cup wheat flour would become 3/4 cup wheat flour and 1/4 cup almond flour). Or, if it's all or nothing for your recipe, remember to increase the amount of rising agent (by about 1/2 teaspoon per cup of almond flour added) to account for the extra weight.

6. Avocado puree for butter

They're both fats (albeit very different fats) and have nearly the same consistency at room temperature. The creaminess and subtle flavor of the avocado lend itself well to the texture of fudge brownies and dark chocolate flavorings. It can take some experimenting to get this swap perfect, but generally, using 1 cup of avocado puree per cup of butter works.

7. Brown rice cereal with flax meal for Rice Crispies

Brown puffed rice has the same texture as conventional white rice, but with half the calories. The flax adds extra fiber, omega-3 fatty acids and phytochemicals to the mix without compromising flavor!

8. Marshmallow Fluff for frosting

Replacing the fat and sugar in frosting with marshmallow achieves the perfect consistency with many fewer calories. While two tablespoons of marshmallow have just 40 calories and 6 grams of sugar (and no fat), the same amount of conventional frosting can pack up to 100 calories, 14 grams of sugar and 5 grams of fat.

9. Natural peanut butter for reduced-fat peanut butter

While they may appear better than traditional Skippy or Jiff, reduced fat versions of peanut butter can actually have more sugar—and an extra-long list of artificial additives—than the classics. Natural peanut butter (preferably unsalted) provides the same sweetness without all the extra junk.

10. Vanilla for sugar

Cutting sugar in half and adding a teaspoon of vanilla as a replacement can give just as much flavor with significantly fewer calories. Assuming the recipe originally calls for one cup of sugar, that's already almost 400 calories cut out! You can't sub this one in equal ratios, but next time you're whipping up some cookies, try cutting 2 tablespoons of sugar and adding an extra 1/2 teaspoon of vanilla extract.

11. Mashed bananas for fats

The creamy, thickening-power of mashed (ripe) banana acts the same as avocado in terms of replacing fat in baking recipes. The consistency is ideal, and the bananas add nutrients like potassium, fiber and vitamin B6. One cup of mashed banana works perfectly in place of 1 cup of butter or oil!

12. Nut flours for flour

A word of caution: Nut flours don't rise the same way as wheat flour so an additional rising agent might be needed when replacing more than ¼ cup of wheat. Many gluten-free blogs detail how to streamline nut flour-based baking. And while these flours are typically higher in calories and fat, they also have more fiber and protein. Nut flours do tend to be heavier than classic wheat, so make sure to up the amount of baking powder and baking soda in the recipe so the dough can rise as normal. Another option is to replace only part of the flour in a recipe with nut flour!

13. Coconut flour for wheat flour
High in fiber and low in carbohydrates, coconut flour is a great partial substitute for wheat flour in baking recipes. Be careful, though—using more than half a cup at a time could allow the flour's bitterness to take over. Substitutes can be tricky in baking, so when using coconut flour, be sure to add an equal amount of extra liquid! In baked goods, you generally want to substitute only 1/4 to 1/3 cup of coconut flour for 1 cup of wheat flour.

14. Meringue for frosting
Made from just egg whites and sugar, meringue can be a great fat-free substitution for traditional frosting. Feel like going a step further? Take a torch to it. Lightly charring the edges of the meringue can add a nice caramelized flavor. (Not to mention a cool visual effect!)

15. Graham crackers for cookies (in pie crusts)
Who doesn't love a freshly baked cookie-crust pie? Next time, refrain from the traditional sugar or Oreo cookie crust and grab the reduced-fat graham crackers.

Reduced-fat graham crackers offer the same consistency and flavor with about half the calories of the conventional options.

16. Evaporated skim milk for cream

It's the same consistency with a fraction of the fat. Evaporated milk tends to have a bit more sugar (only about 2 grams), but the major drop in fat content is well worth the switch. This substitute is an even swap, too (1 cup cream = 1 cup evaporated milk)!

17. Stevia for sugar

The natural sweetener stevia is lower in calories and up to 300 times sweeter than sugar. But watch the grocery bill—this fashionable sweetener can also cost up to 5 times as much as granulated sugar. Since it's so much sweeter, swap with caution: A recipe calling for 1 cup of sugar should be swapped for 1 teaspoon liquid stevia (or about 2 tablespoons stevia powder).

18. Prunes for butter

In brownies and other dark baked goods, prune puree makes for a perfect butter substitute while cutting more than half the calories and fat. Combine 3/4 cup prunes with 1/4 cup boiling water and puree to combine. Sub in equal amounts in most dark baked good recipes.

19. Cacao nibs for chocolate chips

News flash: Those chocolate chips actually start out as cacao nibs–the roasted bits of cocoa beans that then get ground down and turned in to chocolate. Opting for these unprocessed (or at least less processed) morsels cuts out the additives and added sugar in chocolate, while also delving out a healthy dose of antioxidants.

20. Chia seeds for butter

These funny-lookin' little seeds are good for more than just growing countertop pets. Combine 1 tablespoon chia seeds with 9 tablespoons of water. Let sit for 15 minutes and you get a gel that's the perfect consistency to stand in for fat in baking recipes. One word of caution: don't try to cut out all the fat with this substitute–it works best when subbing an equal amount of this mixture for half of the fat in a recipe.

21. Chia seeds for eggs

Surprise! Combining 1 tablespoon chia seeds with 1 cup of water left to sit for 15 minutes yields a perfect 1-

to-1 egg substitute for baking. (But we probably wouldn't suggest subbing chia for butter and eggs in the same recipe!)

22. Flax meal for eggs

This one's an old vegan trick. Mix 1 tablespoon ground flax seeds (aka flax meal) with 3 tablespoons of warm water and whisk with a fork to combine. Now let it sit in the fridge for 5-10 minutes before subbing for 1 egg in any baked recipe.

Smarter Carbs

23. Brown rice for white rice

When white rice is processed, the "brown" bran layer gets stripped away, cutting out essential nutrients (like fiber). Opt for brown rice for a fuller nutritional profile.

24. Quinoa for couscous

While couscous is made from processed wheat flour, quinoa is a whole-grain superfood packed with protein and nutrients. Bonus points: They have almost the exact same texture.

25. Zucchini ribbons for pasta
Thin strips or ribbons of zucchini are a great stand-in for carb-packed pasta.

26. Turnip mash for mashed potatoes
While one cup of mashed potatoes made with whole milk racks up about 180 calories (and that's before the inevitable salt and butter), a cup of mashed turnip (which doesn't need milk or butter to get that creamy consistency) has only 51 calories. Add some fresh herbs in place of salt and it's a much healthier stand-in for the classic mash.

27. Grated steamed cauliflower for rice
Cut both calories and carbs with this simple switch. The texture is virtually the same, as is the taste.

28. Mashed cauliflower for mashed potatoes
Just like the turnip mash, mashed cauliflower has only a fraction of the calories of potatoes and it's nearly impossible to taste the difference. Got picky eaters at the table? Try mixing half potato, half cauliflower.

29. Rolled oats for breadcrumbs

While breadcrumbs can pack extra sodium, using rolled oats seasoned with herbs is a great way to sneak another whole grain into any meal.

30. Whole wheat pasta for regular pasta

Just as with bread, whole wheat pasta beats regular pasta with higher fiber content and about 50 fewer calories per serving (depending on the brand).

31. Crushed flax or fiber cereal for bread crumbs

Crushing a fiber-rich cereal and mixing it with some herbs makes an easy lower-sodium substitution for traditional breadcrumbs.

32. Spaghetti squash for pasta

Roasted and pulled apart with a fork, spaghetti squash is a great low-carb and lower-calorie substitute for pasta. One squash will make between two and three servings.

33. Pita for bread

One 4-inch whole-wheat pita runs around 80 calories and only 1 gram of fat (though there is some variation from brand to brand). Two slices of whole-wheat bread typically come in at around 138 calories!

34. Lettuce leaves for tortilla wraps
It's not a perfect swap, but forgoing the carbs for fresh lettuce is a fun (and easy) switch that can lighten up any wrap or taco dish.

35. Corn tortilla for flour tortilla
Half the calories and fat.

36. Whole wheat bread for white bread
You've heard it all before, but it's just that important! Whole-grain wheat beats out processed white with a complete nutrition profile and better flavor and texture.

37. Quinoa for oatmeal
Cooked with milk (cow, almond, hemp) and some cinnamon, quinoa makes a perfect protein-packed hot breakfast.

38. Steel-cut oatmeal for instant oatmeal
Chewy and a little crunchy, these guys are nothing like their instant oatmeal cousins. While rolled oats are—

literally–rolled into a flat grain, steel cut oats are diced whole grains that maintain more of their fiber-rich shell. Rich in B vitamins, calcium, and protein, steel-cut oats also lack the added sugar that often comes with instant varieties.

Healthier Proteins

39. Dry beans for canned beans
Canned beans are convenient, sure, but they also tend to have excess sodium and plenty of preservatives. Plus, even though the canned versions are dirt cheap, dried beans are even cheaper! It may take a little more work (just some simple soaking and boiling), but this switch is still well worth it.

40. Prosciutto or pancetta for bacon
Bacon is often the go-to for that smoky flavor in savory dishes (and even in some sweet ones). But opting for a few slices of prosciutto or pancetta can help cut both calories and fat. While bacon has about 70 calories and 6 grams of fat for two slices, prosciutto has just 30 calories and 4 grams in an equally weighted sample.

41. Two egg whites for one whole egg
One egg yolk holds more than half the recommended daily cholesterol for the average adult. Trading out the yolk for a second white will cut out the cholesterol while doubling the protein. If making a dish that requires more eggs, keep one to two yolks for their rich vitamins A, E, D, and K content, but consider swapping out the rest.

42. White-meat, skinless poultry or dark-meat poultry
The biggest chicken debate to date: white meat vs. dark meat. And the white meat has it beat—lower in calories and fat, higher in protein and iron.

43. Egg Beaters for egg yolks
A solid substitution for many egg dishes (like omelets or frittatas)—and even for something more complicated, like Hollandaise sauce.

44. Bison for beef
Higher in B vitamins and lower in fat, bison is a great beef substitute.

45. Ground turkey for ground beef

Ground turkey (or chicken) is a great substitute for ground beef to cut down on saturated fat and calories. Reminder: Because of the lower fat content, ground poultry often ends up drier than beef, but a few tablespoons of chicken stock can solve the problem in a snap!

46. Quinoa and ground turkey for rice and ground beef (in stuffed peppers)

More protein and antioxidants in the quinoa and less fat in the ground turkey make this an all-around healthier option for this popular side dish.

Snacks, Sides & Sweets

47. Veggies for pita (as a dipping tool)

Forget the pita. Fresh veggies work as killer dippers with hummus and contain both fewer carbs and more vitamins.

48. Cauliflower puree for egg yolks (in deviled eggs)

For that devilish Southern favorite—deviled eggs—try replacing half the yolks in the filling with cauliflower puree. The taste remains the same, as does the texture, but without the extra dose of cholesterol.

49. Plain yogurt with fresh fruit for flavored yogurt
Pre-flavored yogurts often come packed with extra sugar. To skip the sugar rush without sacrificing flavor, opt for plain yogurt (or better yet, plain Greek Yogurt) and add fresh fruit and/or honey or agave for a hint of sweetness.

50. Arugula, romaine, spinach, and/or kale for iceberg lettuce
All greens are not created equal. Darker greens usually mean more nutrients like iron, vitamin C, and antioxidants.

51. Frozen or fresh fruits for canned fruit
Cut down on excess sugar and preservatives by choosing fresh or frozen varieties.

52. Edamame hummus for regular hummus
While hummus might look innocent from the sidelines, it can be a danger-food because it's packed with more than 50 calories in two tablespoons. That's why switching to an

edamame-based hummus can help reduce the danger (fat and calories) while still providing a delicious dip.

53. *Kale chips for potato chips*

Who would've guessed that a leafy-green could make such delicious chips? When lightly tossed in olive oil and some seasoning (salt and pepper, paprika, or chili powder work well) and baked, these curly greens turn into a delightfully delicate crunchy snack with less fat than the classic fried potato chip.

54. *Dark chocolate for M&Ms (in trail mix)*

The problem with most trail mixes? They pack in the sugar-filled, candy-coated chocolate and dried fruit. Instead, make your own trail mix with unsalted nuts and dark chocolate bits (lower in sugar), which are high in free-radical-fighting flavonoids—a benefit that completely outweighs that candy-coated sweetness.

55. *Popcorn for potato chips*

Lower in calories and fat, natural popcorn without pre-flavored seasonings is a great snack alternative to replace those oily, super-salty potato chips. Try made-at-home flavors by adding cinnamon, chili powder, or Parmesan.

56. Banana ice cream for ice cream

No milk, no cream, no sugar... but the same, delicious consistency. It's easy! Just freeze bananas, then puree.

57. Sweet potato fries for French fries

Opting for sweet potatoes rather than the traditional adds an extra dose of fiber and vitamins A, C and B6. Plus, it cuts out roughly 20 grams of carbohydrates per one-cup serving. Just don't overdo it!

58. Frozen yogurt for ice cream

Picking frozen yogurt over ice cream can help cut down fat content!

Condiments & Sauces

59. Coconut milk for cream

Coconut milk is a great substitute for heavy cream in soups and stews. And don't be turned off by the word "coconut"—it doesn't taste like the sweetened shredded kind!

60. Greek yogurt for sour cream

Half the fat and calories, yet the taste and texture are virtually identical. Plus, nonfat Greek yogurt offers an extra dose of lean protein.

61. Greek yogurt for mayo (in tuna/chicken salad)

Add some herbs and a squeeze of lemon juice, and they'll taste almost identical. Plus, this swap will save on calories and fat, and provide an extra dose of protein.

62. Nutritional yeast for cheese

The taste and texture are a little bit different, but the creamy goodness is pretty comparable. Instead of topping that taco with cheddar, try a sprinkle of nutritional yeast for a cheesy flavoring with much less fat.

63. Nuts for croutons (in salads)

Every salad needs that extra crunch. But rather than getting the extra carbs (and often fat and sodium) that come with croutons, try some lightly toasted slivered almonds, pecans or walnuts.

64. *Avocado mash for mayo*

Half a mashed avocado is a great substitute for mayo on any sandwich. Both give some moisture, but avocado packs a big dose of vitamin E and cholesterol-checking monosaturated fat. And while a typical two-tablespoon serving of mayonnaise has about 206 calories and 24 grams of fat, half an avocado has only 114 calories and 10.5 grams of fat.

65. *Sliced tomatoes for tomato sauce (on pizza)*

Cut out the extra sodium, sugar and preservatives by replacing jarred tomato sauce with fresh sliced tomatoes. The texture is a bit different, but the flavor is much more vibrant and fresh!

66. *Low-fat cottage cheese for sour cream*

They both add a creamy texture to many dishes, but sour cream is packed with fat while low-fat cottage cheese is packed with protein.

67. *Pureed fruit for syrup*

Whether it's to sweeten flapjacks or a nice whole-wheat waffle, pureed fruit warmed on the stovetop with a bit of honey packs much less sugar than classic maple. Plus, it provides an extra dose of antioxidants and vitamins.

68. Herbs or citrus juice

Food doesn't need to be salted to taste good! Fresh herbs and citrus juice can provide just as much flavor without the added risks of excess sodium intake.

69. Garlic powder for salt

Just like fresh herbs, garlic powder can provide a flavorful-punch without adding sodium. A word of caution, don't mistake garlic powder for garlic salt.

70. Low-sodium soy sauce for standard soy sauce

The taste is virtually the same, but choosing a low or reduced-sodium variety can cut down sodium intake by nearly half.

71. Homemade salad dressing for bottled dressing

By making dressing from scratch at home, it's easy to cut out the added sugar, sodium, and preservatives typically found in pre-made dressings. Try mixing vinegar or lemon juice and oil in a 2:1 ratio and flavoring with spices like rosemary, thyme, oregano and pepper!

Drinks & Alcohol

72. Seltzer water with citrus slice instead of soda
Instead of sugary sodas, opt for a glass of sparkling water with a few slices of citrus–grapefruit, lime, orange and lemon all work well–for a little extra flavor.

73. Skim milk for whole or 2% milk
Fewer calories and fat with the same amount of protein makes this switch well worth it.

74. Cinnamon for cream and sugar (in coffee)
Cutting out the cream and sugar in favor of a sprinkle of cinnamon can cut up to 70 calories per cup. Plus, cinnamon can boost metabolism.

75. Unsweetened iced tea for juice or bottled teas
While delicious and convenient, bottled teas, juices, and sports drinks are packed with sugar and calories. When in the mood for something icy with a little flavor, opt for a home-brewed, unsweetened iced tea.

76. Americano for latte

Just by cutting the milk out of that daily latte in favor of hot water, the calorie count drops by more than 150. It's a smart switch, especially by the fourth or fifth cup.

77. Red wine for white wine

While white wine is usually lower in calories, red offers health benefits unmatched by the white stuff, including cancer-fighting compounds and natural cholesterol checks.

78. Soda water for juice (as a mixer)

Rum and coke. Cranberry and vodka. Sure, these sugary mixers take care of the inner sweet tooth. But try mixing liquor with soda water and a slice of fruit (or even just a splash of juice) and down goes the sugar (and calorie) count.

79. Soda water for tonic water

Yes, it's clear and bubbly, just like soda water, but tonic water is actually full of sugar. Adding plain soda water and a pinch of lime gives almost the same taste with 32 grams less sugar per 12 ounces.

Cooking Tips

80. Olive oil spray for olive oil from the bottle
Using a spray bottle is a great way to cut down on oil while still getting the non-stick benefits. A little mist is all that's needed!

81. Olive oil for butter
When cooking eggs, this simple switch is a great way to cut down on saturated fats while getting a healthy dose of essential omega-3 fatty acids.

82. Oven or pan-frying for deep frying
Yes, those chicken tenders are deliciously greasy, but by foregoing the oil bath for just a misting of oil in a pan or oven, it's easy to cut fat without sacrificing flavor.

83. Steaming for boiling
While both are great options for meats and veggies, steaming is king because it removes fewer nutrients from vegetables. While boiling can leech out some of the better nutrients (hence why water turns green after boiling broccoli), steaming keeps all that green goodness inside the veggies.

ZONDRA'S FAVORITE RECIPES!

If possible, always use USDA Certified Organic Ingredients

Tangy Mango Dip

Ingredients:

- 6 tablespoons light cottage cheese
- 1/4 cup sun-dried tomatoes in olive oil, drained well
- 1/4 cup light cream cheese
- 1 teaspoon fresh lemon juice
- Dash garlic powder
- Dash hot sauce (optional)
- 2 - 4 tablespoons buttermilk
- Baked potato chips

Directions:

1. In a food processor, combine the cottage cheese, sun-dried tomatoes, cream cheese, lemon juice, garlic powder and hot sauce if using. Pulse until mixture forms a slightly textured dip, adding buttermilk to thin as desired.

2. Scrape mixture into a bowl and serve with baked potato chips. The dip will keep in the refrigerator up to two days.

Nutrition Information:

Servings Per Recipe: 6
Per Serving: 162 cal., 5 g total fat (2 g sat. fat), 23 g carb. (2 g fiber), 5 g pro.

Fish Sticks

Ingredients:

- Canola oil cooking spray
- 1 cup whole-wheat dry breadcrumbs or ½ cup plain dry breadcrumbs
- 1 cup whole-grain cereal flakes
- 1 teaspoon lemon pepper
- ½ teaspoon garlic powder
- ½ teaspoon paprika
- ¼ teaspoon salt
- ½ cup all-purpose flour
- 2 large egg whites, beaten

- 1 pound wild-caught tilapia fillets, cut into ½-by-3-inch strips

Directions:

- Prepare: 30 m
- Ready In: 40 m

1. Preheat oven to 450°F. Set a wire rack on a baking sheet; coat with cooking spray.
2. Place breadcrumbs, cereal flakes, lemon pepper, garlic powder, paprika and salt in a food processor or blender and process until finely ground. Transfer to a shallow dish.
3. Place flour in a second shallow dish and egg whites in a third shallow dish. Dredge each strip of fish in the flour, dip it in the egg and then coat all sides with the breadcrumb mixture. Place on the prepared rack. Coat both sides of the breaded fish with cooking spray.
4. Bake until the fish is cooked through and the breading is golden brown and crisp. About 10 minutes.

Spinach Orange Green Smoothie

Ingredients:

- 1 navel orange, peeled
- 1/2 banana, peeled
- 1 cup tightly packed spinach
- 1/4 cup coconut water, adjusted as desired
- 1 tablespoon hemp seeds, optional
- Ice

Directions:

1. Blend until nice and creamy!

Serves 1

Healthy Meatloaf

Ingredients:

- cooking spray
- 1 tablespoon olive oil
- 1 green bell pepper, diced
- 1/2 cup diced sweet onion

- 1/2 teaspoon minced garlic
- 1 pound extra-lean (95%) ground beef
- 1 cup whole wheat bread crumbs
- 2 large eggs
- 3/4 cup shredded carrot
- 3/4 cup shredded zucchini
- salt and ground black pepper to taste
- 1/4 cup ketchup, or to taste
- Add all ingredients to list

Directions:

- Prep: 15 m
- Cook: 45 m
- Ready In: 1 h

1. Preheat oven to 400 degrees F (200 degrees C). Spray a 9x5-inch loaf pan with cooking spray.
2. Heat olive oil in a skillet over medium heat; cook and stir green bell pepper and onion in the hot oil until onion is transparent and bell pepper is softened, 5 to 10 minutes. Add garlic and cook until fragrant, 1 to 2 minutes.

3. Combine ground beef, bread crumbs, eggs, carrot, zucchini, salt, pepper, and bell pepper mixture in a large bowl; mix well using your hands. Press meat mixture into the prepared loaf pan.

4. Bake in the preheated oven until no longer pink in the center, 35 to 40 minutes. An instant-read thermometer inserted into the center should read at least 160 degrees F (70 degrees C). Spread ketchup on the top of the meatloaf and continue baking until bubbling, about 5 minutes more.

Tip:

- Aluminum foil helps keep food moist, ensures it cooks evenly, keeps leftovers fresh, and makes clean-up easy.

Nutrition Facts:

Per Serving: 377 calories; 20.1 g fat; 24 g carbohydrates; 26.4 g protein; 157 mg cholesterol; 457 mg sodium.

Orange Salmon

Ingredients:

- 2 oranges, sliced into rounds
- 1 onion, thinly sliced
- 1 1/2 tablespoons olive oil
- 5 (6 ounce) salmon fillets
- 1 tablespoon lemon pepper
- 1 1/2 teaspoons garlic powder
- 1 tablespoon dried parsley
- 1/2 cup orange juice
- 1 1/2 tablespoons lemon juice
- 1 tablespoon honey

Directions:

- Prep: 15 min
- Cook: 40 min
- Ready In: 55 min

1. Preheat the oven to 400 degrees F (200 degrees C).
2. In a small bowl or cup, stir together the lemon pepper, garlic powder, and dried parsley. Place the

slices from one of the oranges in a single layer in the bottom of a 9x13 inch baking dish. Place a layer of onion slices over the orange. Drizzle with a little bit of olive oil, and sprinkle with half of the herb mixture.

3. Place the dish in the preheated oven, and roast for about 25 minutes, or until the onions are browned and tender. Remove the dish from the oven, and increase the temperature to 450 degrees F (220 degrees C).

4. Push the onion and orange slices to the outer edge of the baking dish, and place the salmon fillets in the center. Season with the remaining half of the herb mixture. Whisk together the orange juice, lemon juice and honey in a small bowl. Pour evenly over the salmon.

5. Bake for 12 to 15 minutes in the preheated oven, or until the salmon is opaque in the center. Remove fillets to a serving dish, and discard the roasted orange. Garnish fillets with roasted onions and fresh orange slices.

Nutrition Facts:

Per Serving: 345 calories; 14.9 g fat; 17.4 g carbohydrates; 34.7 g protein; 93 mg cholesterol; 353 mg sodium.

Slow-Roasted Char with Fennel Salad

Ingredients:

- ½ cup unseasoned rice vinegar
- 1 tablespoon sugar
- 1 teaspoon caraway seeds
- 2 teaspoons kosher salt, plus more
- 6 garlic cloves, thinly sliced
- 1 small fennel bulb, thinly sliced on a mandoline, divided
- 1¼ pounds arctic char or salmon fillet
- 4 tablespoons olive oil, divided
- Freshly ground black pepper
- 1 tablespoon fresh lemon juice
- 1 tablespoon chopped preserved lemon peel
- ½ cup dill fronds

Directions:

1. Preheat oven to 300°. Bring vinegar, sugar, caraway seeds, 2 tsp. salt, and ⅓ cup water in a small saucepan to a simmer over medium heat, stirring to dissolve sugar. Remove from heat and add garlic. Let sit until garlic is slightly softened, 10–15 minutes.

2. Add half of fennel and toss to coat. Let sit until fennel softens slightly and tastes pickled, 8–10 minutes.

3. Meanwhile, place char in a 2 or 3 qt. baking dish and coat with 1 tbsp. olive oil; season with salt and pepper. Roast until flesh easily flakes apart and a paring knife inserted into fish meets no resistance, 15–18 minutes.

4. Drain fennel mixture; discard liquid. Toss in a small bowl with lemon juice, preserved lemon, remaining 3 tbsp. oil and remaining fennel; season with salt and pepper. Mix in dill.

5. Serve char topped with fennel salad.

6. Do Ahead: Garlic and fennel can be pickled 1 day ahead. Cover and chill.

Low-Fat Baked Chicken

Ingredients:

- 4 skinless, boneless chicken breasts
- 4 cups plain non-fat yogurt
- 2 cups cornflakes cereal

Directions:

1. Preheat oven to 350 degrees F (175 degrees C).
2. Crush the cornflake crumbs between 2 pieces of wax paper.
3. Dip the chicken breasts in the yogurt, coating both sides. Roll in crushed cornflake crumbs to coat all sides, then place in a 9x13 inch baking dish. Bake the chicken in the preheated oven for 30 minutes.

Nutrition Facts:

Per Serving: 280 calories; 1.5 g fat; 31.2 g carbohydrates; 38.2 g protein; 73 mg cholesterol; 313 mg sodium.

Asian Chicken Salad

Ingredients:

For the dressing:
- 1 teaspoon minced garlic
- 1/4 cup reduced-sodium soy sauce
- 2 tablespoons rice vinegar
- 1 1/2 tablespoons honey
- Pinch of ground ginger

For the salad:
- 1 cup cooked chicken breast, chopped or shredded
- 1 cup shelled edamame beans, cooked according to packaged directions and cooled
- 2 medium bell peppers, diced
- 1 cup shredded carrots
- 4 cups tricolore coleslaw mix
- 1/2 cup chopped cilantro
- 3 green onions, chopped, optional
- 1/4 cup toasted almonds, optional
- 1 tablespoon sesame seeds, optional

Directions:

1. Mix the garlic, soy sauce, rice vinegar, honey, and ginger in a small bowl to make the dressing.
2. Place the chicken, edamame, bell peppers, carrots and coleslaw mix in a large bowl. Toss to combine.
3. Add the dressing to the salad and combine until the salad is fully coated. Add the cilantro and mix again.
4. Sprinkle the green onions, toasted almonds, and sesame seeds on top, if desired.
5. Serve immediately, or let it chill for the best taste possible.

Japanese Style Green Beans

Ingredients:

- 1 tablespoon canola oil
- 1 1/2 teaspoons sesame oil
- 1 pound fresh green beans, washed
- 1 tablespoon soy sauce
- 1 tablespoon toasted sesame seeds

Directions:

- Prep 5 minutes
- Cook 15 minutes
- Ready in 20 minutes

Warm a large skillet or wok over medium heat. When the skillet is hot, pour in canola and sesame oils, then place whole green beans into the skillet. Stir the beans to coat with oil. Cook until the beans are bright green and slightly browned in spots, about 10 minutes. Remove from heat, and stir in soy sauce; cover, and let sit about 5 minutes. Transfer to a serving platter, and sprinkle with toasted sesame seeds.

Nutrition Facts:

Per Serving: 97 calories; 6.6 g fat; 8.9 g carbohydrates; 2.7 g protein; 0mg cholesterol; 233 mg sodium.

DO IT YOURSELF SKIN CARE TREATMENTS!

Be sure to use USDA certified organic ingredients whenever possible

Parsley Eye Mask

What you need:
A handful of parsley
1 tablespoon hot water

How to:

Roughly chop the parsley and drop it into a small bowl. Grind the leaves with the back of a wooden spoon (or drop them into a food processor if you're short on time). Add the hot water and stir the mixture together. When it has cooled, soak up the juice into two cotton balls or pads. Lie down on your back and gently press the cotton balls under your eyes for 10 minutes.

Why it works:

Parsley contains vitamin C, chlorophyll, and vitamin K --

ingredients that help lighten skin (think: dark under-eye circles) and reduce puffiness.

Cucumber Cooling Mask

(Best for: Irritated and/or breakout prone skin)
What you need:
1 cucumber, peeled and sliced
1 teaspoon honey

How to:

Start by pureeing the cucumber pieces in a food processor. Add the puree into a bowl and mix in the honey with a spoon. Lie on your back (with a towel under your head, in case the mask drips a little); massage the mixture all over your face, making a circular motion with your fingertips. Let the mask sit on your skin for 10 minutes before rinsing off with lukewarm water.

Why it works:

The vitamin C in cucumbers is a natural antioxidant that soothes irritated skin, while reducing puffiness and swelling.

Sea Salt Foot Scrub

Get rid of rough, dry skin with this easy salt foot scrub. Choose your favorite essential oil and mix with coarse sea salt. All it takes is a simple soak and your feet will be ready for summer sandals.

How to:

Use 2 to 3 tablespoons of coarse sea salt per gallon of water. Add in a few dabs of your

favorite therapeutic quality essential oil. Relax and soak!

Why it works:

Salt helps ease pain and stiffness in the joints. It naturally exfoliates skin, sloughing

away dead skin cells.

Chocolate-Oatmeal Face Mask

Best for: Sun-damaged complexion

What you need:

1/3 cup cocoa

1/4 cup honey

2 tablespoons heavy cream or sour cream

3 tablespoons old-fashioned oatmeal (powdered in a food processor)

How to:

Use a spoon to mix all of the ingredients together in a bowl until well-blended. With fingers or a fan paintbrush (which you can get from an art supply store), apply the mask onto your face. Use the tips of your fingers to massage the mask into the skin. Let the mask work its magic for 15 minutes before rinsing off with lukewarm water.

Why it works:

Cocoa powder is a natural antioxidant that protects skin from UV damage. Oatmeal is a gentle exfoliator and honey is a great antibacterial ingredient.

Tomato Scrub

What you need:

1 medium tomato

1 tablespoon extra virgin olive oil

2 tablespoons salt

How to:

Scoop the flesh out of the tomato and muddle it in a small bowl with the back of a spoon. Add salt and olive oil and mix until blended. Apply to clean dry skin, letting it soak in for at least five minutes. Leftovers? You can keep them refrigerated for a few days.

Why it works:
Tomato and olive oil work together to boost skin's elasticity, while salt sloughs away dead skin cells.

Foot Soak and Detox

What you need:
1 cup epsom salt
1 cup baking soda
1 cup sea salt
¼ cup vinegar
1 cup warm water
3 drops of peppermint oil

How to:
Pamper your feet by mixing all of the dry ingredients -- salts and baking soda -- in a large bowl or basin. Add the vinegar, water, and peppermint oil, stirring until everything is completely dissolved. Let your feet soak for 20 minutes and then pat dry before applying foot lotion or petroleum jelly.

<u>*Why it works:*</u>
Salt helps ease pain and stiffness in the joints, while naturally exfoliating skin. Baking soda, vinegar, and peppermint oil are deodorizers.

DESK & OFFICE EXERCISES

1. The Twinkle Toe
Tap into your inner Fred Astaire by speedily tapping those toes on the floor under your desk. Or graduate to a harder (and less inconspicuous) move: Stand in front of a small trashcan and lift up those legs to tap the toes on its edge, alternating feet, in soccer-drill fashion.

2. The Stair Master
Want to avoid elevator small talk in favor of elevating the heart rate? Take the stairs! Accelerate on the straight-aways and take two at a time every other flight for a real leg burn.

3. The Slog, Then Jog
Instead of slogging away for hours nonstop, take a mini-break for a stationary jog. Pop up from your chair (admire the butt imprint left behind) and jog in place. Willing to

huff and puff a little more? Pick up those knees! Continue for one minute, return to spreadsheets, and repeat.

4. *The Celebratory Split Squat Jumps*

Win over a new client? Figure out how to un-jam the printer? Is it finally Friday? Celebrate with the split squat jump. With feet hip-width apart, step the left leg back two feet and balance on the ball of the foot. Next, lower into a lunge, and then accelerate upwards in an explosion of celebration. While in the air, switch feet so that the left foot is planted firmly in front and the right leg is now behind. Repeat 10-12 times on each side.

5. *The Cubicle Wanderer*

Walking during work is totally underrated. Take a stroll down the hall to catch up with coworkers or welcome a new employee. Or, instead of dialing extensions and sending lazy emails to the manager two doors down, put in some face time. Just beware of tempting candy jars when making the rounds.

6. *The Mover and Shaker*

Release stress and spark some energy with a quick bout of seated dancing when no one is looking! Salsa anyone?

Legs and Butt

7. The Wall (Street) Sit
Wall sits are great for building strength and endurance. Standing with your back against the wall, bend the knees and slide your back down the wall until the thighs are parallel to the floor. Sit and hold for 30-60 seconds, while browsing the newspaper (or whatever you like to read). For some extra burn, try crossing the right ankle over the left knee, hold for 15 seconds, then switch!

8. The Last Man Standing
Sure, standing around isn't exactly traditional exercise, but research shows it's got more than a leg up on sitting. After all, long periods of sitting are linked to increased risk for diabetes, obesity, and cardiovascular disease, whereas standing significantly increases your daily caloric expenditure. Stand whenever you can, and consider roping in other coworkers to have standing meetings too!

9. The Patient Printer
The boss lady just requested that a 200-page presentation be printed "perfectly." Why lackadaisically stand by the printing pages when you could be sculpting

your calves with calf raises? Standing with feet shoulder-width apart, press up onto the tippy toes, pause at the top, then lower back down. Repeat for three sets of 12-15 reps, or until the printing, faxing, or scanning is done. Ready to level up? Try raising only one leg at a time.

10. The Silent Seat Squeeze

Believe it or not, some exercises can be kept under wraps, and this isometric glutes exercise is one of them. To start toning, simply squeeze the buttocks, hold for 5-10 seconds, and release. Repeat until the agenda wraps up or the glutes tire. The results will be uplifting in more ways than one.

11. The Seated Leg Raiser

When pay raises are nowhere to be seen, consider the leg raise. (Bonus: they're hardly noticeable underneath the desk!) While seated, straighten one or both legs and hold in place for five or more seconds. Then lower the leg(s) back to the ground without letting the feet touch the floor. Repeat (alternating legs if raising them separately) for 15 reps. Underwhelmed? Loop a purse or briefcase strap over the ankle for added weight, or for more of an abs workout, add a crunch.

12. The Desk Squat

Mastered the art of standing around? Add a squat! Start standing with feet together (and the desk chair pushed out of the way). Bend the knees slightly so the thighs are almost parallel to the ground as if sitting in a chair. As you bend, raise the arms straight up or towards the computer screen. Keep the knees together and aligned. Hold for 15 seconds and release. Repeat for 4-6 reps.

13. The Lunch Break Hammy

Strengthen the hamstrings with this standing leg curl. Stand behind your chair and hold onto it for support. Gently kick one foot back, aiming the heel for the top of your thigh. Lower the foot back down and repeat the exercise with the other leg. Do 10 reps, take a bite of your lunchtime sandwich, and then do 10 more.

14. The Grim Reamer

Scope out the office for a ream of paper, or a sealed package of printing paper. While seated, place the stack in between the knees and press legs inward, engaging the inner thighs. Continue squeezing the paper ream in place for 30-60 seconds while sorting through the morning's flood of emails.

Shoulders and Arms

15. *The Cubicle Dip*

Triceps dips can be done almost anywhere, including a cubicle. Using a sturdy desk or a non-rolling chair, sit at the very edge and place hands on either side of the body while gripping the chair's edge. With the feet planted on the floor a step or two away from the desk or chair, straighten up the arms to lift up the body. Next, bend the arms to reach a 90-degree angle so that your body dips down, hold, and re-straighten while keeping the body raised above the chair. Complete 8-10 reps.

16. *The Stapler Curl*

Trusty staplers are always guarded closely, especially the red ones. Seated or standing, take the stapler in one hand with the palm facing upwards. Starting at the thighs, bend the elbow and curl the arm up towards the chest, just like a regular dumbbell biceps curl. Pause momentarily and then lower the stapler back down. Continue for 12-15 reps, then switch. Don't have a weighty stapler? Try using a filled water bottle or a heavy change purse.

17. The Prayer

Whether you're praying for a project extension or for more defined arms, this move has you covered. Seated upright with feet flat on the floor, bring the palms together in front of the chest and push both hands together powerfully until you feel the arm muscles contract. Hold the prayer hands pushed together for 20 seconds. Release and repeat the sequence until you feel a little more zen.

18. The Secret Handshake

Let's make a deal. Sitting up and with feet flat on the floor, clasp hands together as if giving yourself a handshake (with one hand's thumb pointing to the floor and the other pointing to the ceiling). Then pull! Resist the motion of both arms (you should definitely feel this in those biceps). Hold for 10 seconds or more, release, and repeat.

19. The Fist Pump

Received approval from the head honcho for extra vacation days? Time to rock out to your favorite playlist while simultaneously toning the arms. Fist punch into the air like a champ (alternating arms, of course), and continue for 60 seconds or more—or until you realize the boss is right behind you.

20. The Knuckle Sandwich

So the big cheese said no to the promotion and returned your project covered in red ink. To relieve frustration and get a fab arm fix, try shadow boxing to the perfect boxing playlist. Stand (if you can) and throw out a few jabs, hooks and uppercuts in rapid succession (just watch out for computers and co-workers). Continue for a minute or longer to blow off steam and tone the arms, chest and core.

21. The Flapper

Whether you've got a thing for the 1920's or enjoy mimicking penguins, this move is for you. Standing with arms by your sides and palms facing behind, pulse the arms backward for 5 seconds. Release and repeat for 12-15 reps. For best results, make sure to keep the arms long and straight!

22. The Casual Lean

Waiting in the hall for a meeting to start? Perfect time to nonchalantly work out the upper arms! Casually leaning against the nearest wall, support your body with the forearm only. Now lean into the wall until the upper arm almost touches it, and then push back out. Repeat for 15 reps. Switch sides.

23. The Lumberjack

While this lumberjack may be wearing slacks instead of plaid, he can still get a good midday workout. Stand and clasp the hands together, resting them on the right shoulder as if holding an axe. Gently swing the imaginary "axe" by straightening the elbows and moving the hands toward the left thigh. Next, bring the clasped hands to the left shoulder followed by a swing to the right thigh. Repeat 15 times on each side.

24. The Office Genie

Want to add a little magic to the workday? Raise the legs into a criss-cross applesauce position while seated in a chair. With your hands on the armrests, push upwards to raise the body off the seat and remain floating for 10-20 seconds. Release back down to the chair, rest for a minute, and repeat. Craving more magic? Try this balancing act while in a chair that spins. Be careful!

Chest, Back, and Neck

25. The Pencil Pinch

Lose the pencil behind the ear. The really suave workers hold it in between their shoulder blades! Show off your traps by rolling back the shoulders until the shoulder blades are pinched together. Pretend you're holding a pencil between the scapulas (or try it for real). Hold for 5-10 seconds, release, and repeat for 12-15 reps.

26. The Shoulder Shrug

Not recommended for board meetings. Simply raise both shoulders up toward the ears, hold for 5 seconds, then relax. Repeat for 15 reps. Feeling unstoppable? Try advanced shoulder shrugs while standing and holding a paper ream in each hand.

27. The Pinstripe Push-Up

This slightly modified wall push-up is more suitable for suits. Standing one to two feet from a sturdy wall (not a cubicle divider), lean forward until palms are flat against the wall, with arms straight and parallel to the ground. Next, bend the elbows to bring the body towards the wall, hold for two seconds, then push back to the starting position. Complete 12-15 reps.

28. The Nape Shaper

Turtleneck season is over—it's time to tone that neck! For the first isometric neck strengthening trick, put your head in your hands as if exasperated by the workday (you may already be in this position - LOL) and press your palms into your forehead as if trying to push the head backward. Resist the motion by engaging the neck muscles. Next, clasp the hands behind the back of the head and try to push the head backward, resisting the motion with your hands. Hold each exercise for 5 seconds. Slowly release, rest, and repeat 5 times each.

Core

29. The Desk Chair Swivel

Lucky enough to have a fun swivel chair? Use its twirl to your advantage with this oblique abs fix. Sitting upright and with the feet hovering over the floor, hold the edge of your desk with your fingers and thumb. Next, use the core to swivel the chair from side to side. Swish back and forth for 15 rounds.

30. The "Weeee" Desk Chair Wheel

Go ahead, play with your wheelie chair (everyone wants to). While seated in a chair with wheels, position yourself at arm's length from a desk or table and grasp its edge with your hands. Next, engage the core, raise the feet slightly off the ground, and pull with your arms until the chair slowly rolls forward and your chest touches the desk's edge. Then roll back by pushing away, with the feet still raised. Repeat 20 times, or until you burn holes into the carpet.

31. The Posture Perfecter

Perfect posture is a must for long days at the desk. Practice safe desk ergonomics by adjusting the chair height to make sure the feet, hips, and arms are at 90-degree angles to the floor. Engage the core to keep the back straight throughout the day. No slouching allowed!

32. The Fab Abs Squeeze

This exercise can be covertly executed when walking down the hall or seated during a call. Simply take a deep breath and tighten the abdominal muscles, bringing them in towards the spine as you exhale. Stay squeezed for 5-10 seconds and release. Repeat for 12-15 reps.

33. The "Crunch Time" Crunch

With both elbows on the thighs, try to curl the chest in towards the legs while resisting the movement with the arms. Hold for 10 seconds, release, and repeat 10 times.

The Best Workouts For Women 40 And Over!

As you age, especially when you hit the tender age of 40, you might begin to wonder what this means for your workout program. How should your workout change compared to that of someone in their 20's.

According to some fitness experts, you definitely need to adapt your workout over time due to the changing needs of your body, but contrary to what you might have been told, it doesn't need to change *a whole lot*.

In my opinion, the single best workout option for women in their 40's is going to be a good resistance training program. It's incredibly important for women in this age group to start with a strength training workout. Why? Because women in their 40's are at a higher risk of losing lean muscle mass. You've heard this old principle 'use it or lose it.' If you aren't putting sufficient stress on your muscles as the weeks pass by, slowly you'll grow weaker, which can make everyday activities harder to perform.

Likewise, your lean muscle mass is the most metabolically active tissue in the body, so the more muscle you lose, the slower your resting metabolic rate will become, which can contribute to weight gain.

One of the biggest reasons why women start to gain weight into their 40's and 50's is because they are losing the lean muscle that helped keep their daily calorie burn higher. If you aren't adjusting your food intake to account for this loss of muscle mass, it will result in weight gain.

Additionally, if you are in your 40's and are really looking to transform your body, weight lifting is the way to do it. While cardio training may help you burn fat, weight lifting will help you reshape your physique, adding curves and muscle in all the right places.

Getting Started With Resistance Training

So how can you get started? First, you'll want to select the best exercises to make the most of your time in the gym. Chances are, you're busy and don't have hours to train, so you'll want to get the most 'bang for your buck.'

Compound exercises will work multiple muscle groups at once, help you gain functional strength, and burn the most calories per session. They should be your focus. These include moves such as bench pressing or push-ups, bent over rows, shoulder presses, squats, lunges, deadlifts and pull-ups (or pull-downs).

Focus on these first and foremost, then you can add other exercises such as bicep curls, tricep extensions, lateral raises, leg extensions, and hamstring curls if you'd like.

You should focus on lifting a heavy enough weight that you are fully fatigued by the time you finish around 8-10 reps without losing proper form. This will give you both the strength-training stimulus to help generate more lean muscle mass while keeping your metabolic rate and calorie burn higher.

Finally, rest for a few seconds between sets. You don't want to rest too long or you'll lose some of the metabolic boosting effects this workout provides. At the same time, don't rest so little that you can't challenge yourself with a heavy weight.

To help give you an idea of how to implement this, on the following pages are examples of what a full body workout for women over 40 would look like. Always begin with prayer and a brief five to ten minute warm-up and finish up with prayer and some light stretching at the end.

Full Weight Training Workout For Women Over 40!

- Squats – 3 sets of 8 reps

- Bench Press – 3 sets of 8 reps

- Bent Over Rows – 3 sets of 8 reps

- Leg Press – 3 sets of 10 reps

- Shoulder Press – 3 sets of 10 reps

- Walking Lunges – 2 sets of 12 reps

- Superset* Bicep Curls with Tricep Extensions – 2 sets of 15 reps

- Superset* Lateral Raises with Front Raises – 2 sets of 15 reps

*Note that a superset is performing all the reps of one exercise and then directly moving to the next exercise, doing all the reps of it before taking a rest.

So if you have not yet started with resistance training, lean towards this style of exercise as you formulate your workout plan. It'll serve you very well both in your 40's as well as in the years beyond.

Full Cardiovascular Training Workout For Women Over 40!

Choose any cardio machine, set it on a manual mode (versus pre-set programs), and find your warm-up pace.

For the bulk of the workout, you'll change the settings (incline, speed, resistance, etc.) every few minutes to work at a moderate level, ending with a cool down. Throughout, you'll use the perceived exertion scale, which gauges the intensity at which you're exercising from 1 to 10, to work at the suggested levels.

This workout is really designed just to get an idea of how cardio feels to your body. Feel free to change the settings and adjust it to fit your ability.

- 5 minutes: Warm up at an easy-moderate pace. Perceived Exertion Level (PE): 4

- 5 minutes: Increase speed, incline, and/or resistance so you're just out of your comfort zone but still able to talk. This is your baseline. PE: 5

- 2 minutes: Increase your speed, incline, and/or resistance until you're working a little harder than baseline. PE: 6

- 3 minutes: Reduce your speed, incline, and/or resistance back to baseline. PE: 5

- 1 minute: Increase your speed, incline, and/or resistance until you're working a little harder than baseline. PE: 6

- 4 minutes: Reduce speed, incline, and/or resistance back to a moderate level. PE: 4

Total workout time: 20 minutes

Flexibility Workout

Cardio and strength training may be the cornerstones of any solid workout program, but you don't want to end your workout without stretching. Stretching when your muscles are warm has a number of benefits, from building greater flexibility to offering relaxation and stress relief.

The great thing about stretching is that you don't have to spend a lot of time to get the benefits.

Your First Week

Now that you've gotten an idea of what an exercise routine looks like, it's time to plan your first week of workouts. Here's an idea of how to schedule your cardio and strength-training activity.

Day 1/Monday

Perform the 20 minute cardio routine outlined above, followed by 10 minutes of stretching. 5 minutes before and 5 minutes after your workout. Be sure to pray.

Today's Motivational Scripture:

1 Corinthians 6:19-20 (NIV) *"Do you not know that your bodies are temples of the Holy Spirit, who is in you, whom you have received from God? You are not your own; you were bought at a price. Therefore honor God with your bodies.*

Day 2/Tuesday

For this basic strength training workout, you'll do 1 set of 15 reps of each of the nine exercises listed below, resting briefly between exercises as needed. The workout targets all the muscles in the body, including the chest, shoulders, arms, back, hips, glutes, and thighs. It's short and simple.

It's a great way for beginners to get started with strength training.

- Assisted Lunges

- Modified Push-ups

- Ball Squats

- Overhead Presses

- Dumbbell Rows

- Bicep Curls

- Tricep Extensions

- Crunches on the Ball

- Back Extensions

It's normal to be sore after lifting weights for the first time, or if it's been a long time since you've pumped iron. If you find you're very sore the next day, you might need to take an extra day of rest and back off of your strength workout the next time. Be sure to pray.

Today's Motivational Scripture:

3 John 1-2 (NIV) *"Dear friend, I pray that you may enjoy good health and that all may go well with you, even as your soul is getting along well."*

Day 3/Wednesday

Today you'll do the same 20-minute cardio routine as Day 1, followed by 10 minutes of stretches. 5 minutes before and 5 minutes after your workout.

Today's Motivational Scripture:

1 Corinthians 10:31 NIV) *"So whether you eat or drink whatever you do, do it all for the glory of God."*

Day 4/Thursday

For today's workout, you'll go through the following eight yoga poses holding each for 3 to 5 breaths. Do the workout anytime you like—it will refresh you in the morning and help you unwind before bed. Take your time when performing each exercise and focus on your breath. Breath in and out through the nose, taking the air in through the back of your throat. Do each pose at least once, twice or more if you have time. Be sure to pray.

Today's Motivational Scripture:

1 Timothy 4:8 (NIV) *"For physical training is of some value, but godliness has value for all things, holding promise for both the present life and the life to come.*

- Standing Cat Stretch

- Sun Salutation

- Hanging Back Stretch

- Warrior I

- Warrior II

- Modified Triangle

- Spine Twist

- Corpse Pose

Day 5/Friday

Today's workout involves the basic strength training workout you did on Day 2. As before, perform 1 set of 15 reps for each exercise, resting briefly between moves as needed. If you feel that's too easy, you can always add another set or use heavier weights. Be sure to pray.

Today's Motivational Scripture:

Proverbs 17:22 (NIV) *"A cheerful heart is good medicine, but a crushed Spirit dries up the bones.*

Day 6/Saturday

Today's cardio workout involves interval training which is when you alternate work sets (working at a higher intensity) with rest sets using the perceived exertion scale to monitor your intensity. This workout can be done on any cardio machine.

- 5 minutes: Warm up at an easy pace. PE: 4

- 3 minutes: Rest Set: Increase speed and resistance/ incline to a moderate level.   PE:5

- 1 minute: Work Set: Increase incline and resistance 1 percent to 5 percent to raise the intensity level. PE: 7

- 3 minutes: Rest Set. PE: 5

- 1 minute: Work Set. PE: 7

- 3 minutes: Rest Set. PE: 5

- 5 minutes: Cool down. PE: 4

Today's Motivational Scripture:

Proverbs 31:17 (NIV) *"She sets about her work vigorously; her arms are strong for her tasks.*

Week 1 Recap

- Day 1: 20-Minute Cardio Routine

- Day 2: Basic Strength-Training Workout

- Day 3: 20-Minute Cardio Routine

- Day 4: Basic Yoga

- Day 5: Basic Strength-Training Workout

- Day 6: Beginner Intervals

On Day 1, you completed your first workout. During Week 1, you got through a full week of cardio, strength and flexibility workouts. Now, you're ready to build on that success with progressively more challenging workouts.

That said, keep in mind that the schedules are only suggestions. You may want to do less cardio, more rest days, or you may even want to stick with the same workouts for more than a week. Use this program as a place to start and adjust the schedule so that it works for you.

Week 2

You'll continue with the same schedule as last week (meditating on the same scriptures as well) but progress with a few small changes to keep you challenged.

For cardio, you'll do the same workouts with an added 5 minutes to build endurance and increase your exercise time.

- 5 minutes: Warm up at an easy-moderate pace. Perceived Exertion Level (PE): 4

- 6 minutes: Increase speed, incline, and/or resistance so you're just out of your comfort zone, but still able to talk. This is your baseline. PE: 5

- 3 minutes: Increase your speed, incline, and/or resistance until you're working a little harder than baseline. PE: 6

- 4 minutes: Reduce your speed, incline, and/or resistance back to baseline. PE: 5

- 2 minute: Increase your speed, incline, and/or resistance until you're working a little harder than baseline. PE: 6

- 5 minutes: Reduce speed, incline, and/or resistance back to a moderate level.

Your strength-training workouts include the same exercises, but you'll be doing 2 sets of each for added intensity. Interval training increases by 4 minutes, to 25 minutes.

Modify the workouts as needed to fit your fitness level and goals.

- Day 1: 25-Minute Cardio

- Day 2: Basic Strength Training. Perform each exercise for 2 sets of 15 reps, resting 10 to 30 seconds between sets.

- Day 3: Beginner Intervals - Level 2

- Day 4: Basic Yoga

- Day 5: Basic Strength Training. Perform each exercise for 2 sets of 15 reps, resting 10 to 30 seconds between sets.

- Day 6: 25-Minute Cardio

Week 3

This week, the changes to your workouts are more drastic with higher-intensity cardio workouts, a new and more challenging strength routine, as well as a new yoga workout to try.   Meditate on the same scriptures from week 1.

Your cardio workouts go up from 25 minutes to 30 minutes and the interval workout takes you to higher levels of intensity. The strength routine includes new exercises and heavier weights, and there's a yoga routine performed on an exercise ball, which offers extra support and challenge.

Remember, if these changes feel too fast, keep the same workouts for as long as you need. When they start to feel easy, you'll know you're ready to move on to more challenging workouts.

- Day 1: 30-Minute Cardio

- Day 2: Beginner Total-Body Strength - Level 2. Perform each exercise for 2 set of 15
   reps, resting 10 to 30 seconds between sets.

- Day 3: Beginner Intervals - Level 3

- Day 4: Yoga on the Ball

- Day 5: Beginner Total-Body Strength - Level 2. Perform each exercise for 2 set of 15
  reps, resting 10 to 30 seconds between sets.

- Day 6: 30-Minute Cardio

Week 4

With three weeks of workouts under your belt, you'll maintain your previous schedule with a few small changes to keep things interesting. Meditate on the same scriptures as week 1.

You'll continue with your 30-minute cardio workouts, but try a new interval routine that includes making more frequent changes throughout the workout.

Your strength workout remains the same, but you'll add a second set to challenge your muscles and continue progressing.

- Day 1: 30-Minute Cardio

- Day 2: Beginner Total-Body Strength - Level 2. Perform each exercise for 2 sets of 15 reps, resting 10 to 30 seconds between sets.

- Day 3: Interval Workout - Level 3

- Day 4: Yoga on the Ball

- Day 5: Beginner Total-Body Strength - Level 2. Perform each exercise for 2 sets of 15 reps, resting 10 to 30 seconds between sets.

- Day 6: 30-Minute Cardio

Week 5 - Week 12 and Beyond

To continue making progress, you need to change things up. You will now exercise for 1 hour during each session. Change can come in a variety of ways: You can modify weights, repetitions, intensity, speed, duration, variations on exercises and more. You only have to make one change at a time to see a difference and continue reaching new goals. Meditate on the same scriptures from Week 1.

Our goal is for you to complete 12 weeks or 3 months of our program. During this time, you should notice a drastic change in your mind and body, bringing you closer to your ideal physique and relationship with God. We are as close to God as we choose to be. We are here to help you. I'm so proud of you and this new journey. I know you can do it! Be sure to submit before and after pictures on our facebook page so we can cheer you on as you embark on a new and improved YOU!

Zondra's Prayer!

"Oh Heavenly Father, who has filled the whole earth with beauty. Open our eyes to clearly see Your gracious hand in all Your works. Give every participant of "Faithful, Forty & Fabulously Fit" the mindset and the endurance to complete this 90 day journey for a closer connection to you and a stronger and healthier body. Strengthen me to continue serving You with gladness and thanksgiving. Give me a clean heart. It's because of Your precious Son, Jesus Christ who died on the cross for my sins that I'm not given what I deserve, which is eternal damnation. It is in the precious name of the one who was once dead but is now alive interceding on my behalf that I pray. Thank you

Father for your grace and mercy. In Jesus' precious name I do pray. Amen! Amen! Amen!"

"Stop waiting on someone to help you. Help someone waiting on you."

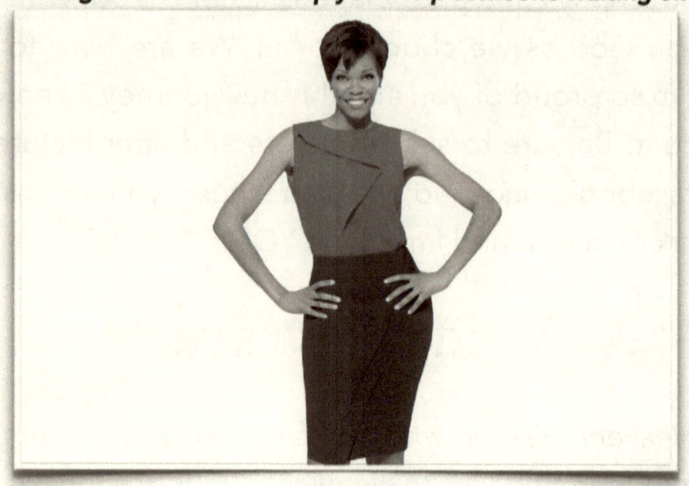

Meet

ZONDRA WILSON

After booking numerous modeling jobs for billion dollar companies such as Merz, Best Buy and Pfizer, Zondra decided to launch a USDA certified organic skin care product line. **"Blu Skin Care, LLC"** manufacturers the only American-made USDA certified organic powdered facial cleanser sold in the United States. Zondra is also the only female, African American owner, manufacturer &

distributor of a skin care company with USDA certified organic accreditation in the United States.

So, why the name **"Blu Skin Care"**? In the Bible, the color blue is sometimes associated with the commandments of God, the importance of remembering them and also the heavenly calling of those who had been chosen by God to be His people (Numbers 15:38-40). Therefore, **"Blu Skin Care"** was the obvious name for the company.

"Blu" prides itself on sourcing the purest and most potent ingredients including organic in all of its formulations.

Our ingredients are plant-derived and formulated with botanicals. We are committed to all of our products being non-GMO as well as nutritious for your skin and as close to 100% USDA certified organic whenever possible.

We promise to support a comprehensive approach in educating people on how to eat right, how to obtain a strong and healthy body and how to get fantastic skin. We encourage you to enjoy a diverse, plant-based diet that provides a full range of nutrients. **"Blu Skin Care, LLC"** relies on foods known to promote health and support recovery from illness and injury. It integrates the very best of both ancient and modern nutritional approaches to form a flexible system of wholeness. At "Blu", we serve the organic skin care industry with the passion and depth of experience that can only come with a lifetime of commitment to the organic movement. We service customers with all skin types.

I enjoy sharing on social media! You can follow me on Instagram @zondrawilson or @bluskincare on Twitter @zondrawilson or @bluskincare and on Facebook @officialzondrawilson or @bluskincare. Also, I encourage you to visit our website at www.bluskincare.info and sign up for our newsletter to get the latest in skin care, valuable coupons and learn of upcoming events!

"WISDOM IS THE PRINCIPAL THING;
THEREFORE GET WISDOM. AND IN ALL YOUR
GETTING, GET UNDERSTANDING." PROV. 4:7(NKJV)

One thing that I would like to share in order to encourage those who are beginning their fitness journeys is that my fitness walk mirrors my walk with God. It is daily, step by step, and consistent. It is very much a walk of faith. I show up and God, well, He's already there to meet me.

Often, I reflect on the first steps of my journey. I was a freshman in high school and Coach Don Gatewood was our school track coach. He approached me one day while I was at football practice. While complimenting my speed, he suggested I try out for the track team.   I actually dodged him for an entire year before I went out for the team. When Coach Gatewood finally convinced me to join, it was one the best decisions I could have made in my life. After the first day of practice, I was our school's newest high hurdler and I loved it. I followed that up by clipping a hurdle and taking a spill in my very first race. Two runners overtook me in the process. I could hear voices in the crowd repeatedly yelling, "get up!" So, I jumped up and chased the two runners down! On sheer determination, I eventually overtook them both and finished my race.

Coach Gatewood was so proud of me but not because I won (I didn't). He was proud of me because I got up and finished the race. I didn't quit in the midst of adversity and walk off of the track when it looked like all was lost. God too, is proud of us when we get back up after a fall. **Proverbs 24:16 (NKJV)** says, "For a righteous man may fall seven times - And rise again, But the wicked shall fall by calamity." In **2 Timothy 4:7 (NKJV)** the Word of God illustrates how He expects us to finish our race and not quit. "I have fought the good fight, I have finished the race, I have kept the faith." In the coming years, I would become a vital part of multiple state championship teams. Additionally, I was named team captain and senior athlete of the year.

When my athletic career concluded I was in the gym sporadically until I got into my late thirties and early forties. During that time, I noticed my peers having various health-related difficulties. Many were overweight or obese accompanied by poor posture. Issues with their knees, back, hips and feet would soon follow at various rates depending on their physical state. Simultaneously, I had strained my lower back while performing simple tasks like tying my shoes on more than one occasion. This became alarming to me because I had never sustained any injuries away from competitive sports. I felt I was "too young" to have this happening to me. It made me feel "old". I had heard all of the horror stories associated with back pain and endless visits to therapists and doctors. Several people I knew endured multiple surgeries directly related to letting their temples go unattended. God revealed to me that every time I stopped training I injured my lower back. During periods of inactivity my body was breaking down. That was my wake up call. If I didn't want to live in pain, I needed to make a change. I unearthed the fire that I had within me when I ran track and began to train without ceasing.

LOVING MY NEIGHBOR AS MYSELF

As my training progressed, God introduced a loving nutritionist and trainer into my life named Maggie. She talked to me about what to put into my body and most importantly, what NOT to put into my body. I had a strong work ethic established from my days of running hurdles but I was missing the nutritional knowledge. Changing my nutrition changed my life! I began to research my food intake on a regular basis. Reading labels became a part of my shopping routine. No longer did I simply toss food items into my cart oblivious to what they contained. Processed foods were eliminated altogether. I learned about the disastrous effects of excess salt and sugar on the body as well as the chemicals being put in our food supply chain. Shortly after improving my diet my body transformed inside and out. I experienced the benefits of proper nutrition almost immediately.

There were unexpected positive consequences of my nutritional shift. They were mental and spiritual. My personal transformation caused me to be more compassionate toward others who were struggling on the outside *and* on the inside. I understood how the physical appearance of an individual most often affected their self-esteem and confidence. Bouts with depression are not uncommon. This understanding cultivated a strong desire within me to encourage and motivate people to set attainable fitness goals and get started on their own personal journey to liberation.

SEEKING HIM FIRST

Multitudes of people have since sought my guidance. I have been humbled by the opportunity to share my experience and knowledge with those that God sends me. The desire I carry to motivate others moved me to start PHREED FITNESS Magazine (www.phreedfitness.com). I sought God for a powerful name that was memorable but didn't sound destructive. My desire is that people be "Phreed" from sickness, disease, depression and other ailments that are products of an unhealthy lifestyle. I desperately wanted to be free. And **John 8:36 (NKJV)** *says that "if the Son sets you free you will be free indeed."*

The fire burning constantly inside of me let me know that God had more in store for me so I prayed about my next step. I was led to enter a national physique competition. Upon entering the Fit Expo in Anaheim, CA, I won 1st place in the 40+ group. This was the culmination of all of my hard work coming to fruition. Several people helped and encouraged me along the way.

It feels so good now to be sharpening my jiu-jitsu skills and working toward my black belt in karate. All of this en route to my dream of getting a role in a superhero-themed film! I'm also booking more fitness photo and video shoots. It is truly awesome to be over forty and feeling better than I did in my twenties! On this journey, I've learned to seek His wisdom in all that I do, whether it be acting in a superhero-themed film, modeling, fitness goals or physique competitions. **James 1: 5-6 (NKJV)** says, *"If any of you lacks wisdom, let him ask of God, who gives to all liberally and without reproach, and it will be given to him. But let him ask in faith, with no doubting, for he who doubts is like a wave of the sea driven and tossed by the wind.* I'm believing and asking in faith, so He will be glorified in my labor. - Keith

HOW TO APPLY!

Daily, pray for Godly wisdom to lead you in every aspect of your life. Pray that you hear His voice clearly for instruction in all that you need to accomplish. God is concerned about what you have been purposed for and He will speak to you. Thank Him and praise Him in advance, giving Him glory for victory in your business, training, and relationships. Worship Him for who He is in the process. Meditate on His Word and listen for His voice.

COMMON HEALTH CONCERNS FOR MEN 40 AND OVER

Before leading you into a training regimen, I wanted to compile a list of concerns that men face going into and beyond middle age. We have to know what we are up against if we are to be successful in our battle against them.

Statistically speaking, men are less likely than women to get routine checkups and to take preventative health measures. Consequently, men procrastinate in the area of personal care until "something" happens and by that time, it's usually too late. My hope and prayer is this; reading the list of health concerns will ignite a fire within you that will cause an effectual change in you and your personal care habits as a man.

As you read this list you will notice that there is a common theme of poor diet and the lack of exercise that contribute to these concerns. They work in concert with age because of the frequency in which they are repeated over the years. Prior to this list are included what I call the "two silent killers" that are hidden in processed foods. Please read on and be edified.

EFFECTS OF SATURATED AND TRANS FAT ON THE BODY

Saturated fat is dietary. Along with trans-fat, saturated fat is unhealthy. Often, they are solid at room temperature. Cheese, butter, red meat, palm and coconut oils have high amounts of saturated fat. Excess saturated fat in your diet over time can lead to heart disease and a host of other health problems.

Our bodies need healthy fats, some of which are outlined for you in this book. Healthy fats provide energy to the body and perform other functions as well. Too much saturated fat can cause cholesterol to build up in the arteries (blood vessels) consequently raising the level of LDL (bad) cholesterol in the body. High cholesterol significantly increases the risk of heart disease and stroke.

Fast foods like pizza, fried foods, and baked goods tend to be high in saturated fat. Eating too much fat will add extra calories to your diet causing you to gain weight. All fats (good or bad) contain 9 calories per gram of fat. This is more than twice as much that is found in carbohydrates and protein. So, you see how this can add up very quickly in our bodies.

Slashing the amount of high-fat foods you eat will help keep your weight in check and your heart healthy. This will significantly reduce your risk for heart disease, the development of diabetes, and other health problems. To assist you in making better health choices, I urge you to start reading the nutritional labels on the foods that you purchase. There is a wealth of information to be gained from them.

THE EFFECTS OF SALT ON THE BODY

Studies overwhelmingly show that excessive salt intake can have devastating effects on our bodies. Salt in excess increases blood pressure by causing your body to hold on to water in an effort to dilute the salt. This results in increased amounts of fluid surrounding the cells within the body and excess fluid in the blood in our bloodstream. Ultimately, this puts a heavier workload on the heart and blood vessels. Over time, this causes blood vessels to stiffen, resulting in high blood pressure, a heart attack or a stroke.

The leading cause of cardio vascular disease is high blood pressure. Two-thirds of strokes and half of heart disease are attributed to high blood pressure. Other areas affected by excessive salt are the kidneys, the brain (dementia) and bones.

It is important to note that our bodies need salt. The recommended amount of salt for a healthy person is 2,300 milligrams per day, but the average American eats about 3,400 milligrams per day. 75 percent of this salt is not added at the table but instead comes from processed or prepared foods. Based on that information, it is safe to say that we need to drastically reduce the amount of processed foods we consume if we are to remain in a healthy state for an extended quality of life.

Below is the list of health concerns I mentioned in paragraph 1 of this section. Read with prudence and with victory in mind.

1. High Cholesterol
   A. Symptoms
      - None – A blood test is the only way to detect
   B. Dangers of high cholesterol include heart disease and stroke
   C. Risk factors
      - Poor diet
      - Saturated fat

- Animal products
  - i. Red meat
  - ii. Full-fat dairy products
- Trans fats
  - i. Commercially baked cookies and crackers
- Obesity
  - i. BMI of 30 or greater
- Large waist circumference
  - i. Men with a waist of 40 inches or more
- Lack of exercise
- Smoking
- Diabetes

D. Prevention
- Eat a low-salt diet that includes fruits, vegetables and whole grains
- Limit the amount of animal fats
- Lose excess weight and maintain a healthy weight
- Quit smoking
- Exercise 30 min. a day
- Alcohol in moderation, if at all

2. Heart Disease
   A. No. 1 cause of death in the United States
   B. The heart ages
      - Healthy diet and exercise reduces the stress on the heart so it's not aging faster than the rest of your body
3. Stroke
   A. The risk of sustaining a stroke doubles each decade after the age of 45
      - Other risk factors
        i. Smoking
        ii. Elevated blood pressure
        iii. Sedentary lifestyle
   B. Leisurely physical activity can slash your stroke risk
4. Elevated Homocysteine (chemical)
   A. 20%-40% of men over 40 have elevated levels of homocysteine (byproduct of digestion)
      - Those with high levels have almost 4 times the risk of suffering a heart attack

- Reduced by avoiding dairy and red meat, exercising, reducing or eliminating alcohol

5. Low Magnesium

   A. Magnesium limits the activity of the cholesterol-converting enzyme

- If it's low we produce more cholesterol than is necessary
- Our soil is magnesium-deficient so we need to supplement

6. Erectile Dysfunction

   A. 30 million Americans

   B. Increases with age

   C. The result of poor circulation and obesity

   D. Forty is the sweet spot

- Prevention includes
  - i. Managing chronic health conditions
  - ii. Stop smoking, limit or avoid alcohol
  - iii. Exercise regularly
  - iv. Reduce stress

7. Prostate Cancer

   A. The risks jump from .005% to 2.2 % in men crossing the threshold of forty

B. There is strong evidence that being overweight or obese increases the risk of advanced prostate cancer

C. Prostate cancer is the second most common cancer among men worldwide. Prostate cancer is more common as men age. In the United States, 97% of all prostate cancers are diagnosed in men 50 years or older.

D. Prevention
- Be a healthy weight, physically active & incorporate a diet rich in whole grains, vegetables, fruits and pulses (legumes) such as beans and lentils
- Limit consumption of:
    i.   "fast foods" and other processed foods high in fat, starches or sugars
    ii. red and processed meat
    iii. sugar sweetened drinks
    iv. alcohol

8. Clogged Arteries

A. Arteries begin to accumulate unwanted deposits called plaques. Plaques can cause inflammation and clogging, eventually leading to other problems .

- Erectile dysfunction
- Heart attacks

B. Prevention

- Add more good fats to your diet. Good fats are also called unsaturated fats. They're found in foods like olives, nuts, avocado, and fish.

- Cut sources of saturated fat, such as fatty meat and dairy. Choose lean cuts of meat, and try eating more plant-based meals.

- Eliminate artificial sources of trans fats. Most artificial trans fats are found in processed, packaged foods like cookies and snack cakes.

- Increase your fiber intake. Soluble fiber helps lower your LDL. You can find soluble fiber in foods like vegetables, lentils, beans, and oats.

- Cut back on sugar. Vitamins and minerals accompany the sugar found naturally in fruit. The sugar found in processed foods like cookies, ice cream, and sugar-sweetened beverages doesn't have nutritional value. Too much added sugar can negatively impact your health.
- Exercise
- Stop Smoking

9. Low Testosterone

A. Testosterone production naturally decreases with age BUT abnormally low levels can lead to fatigue, low sex drive and decreased muscle mass.

B. To increase testosterone levels naturally

- Exercise and lift weights
  i. Weight lifting and high-intensity interval training are the most effective
  ii. New research in obese men suggests that increased physical activity was even

more beneficial than a weight loss diet for increasing testosterone levels

- Eat protein, good fats and carbs
- Minimize stress
- Take vitamin and mineral supplements
- Plenty of rest
- Healthy lifestyle
  i. No excessive alcohol
  ii. No drugs
- Laughter

10. Hypertension (high blood pressure)

A. Can lead to heart attack, stroke, aneurysm, heart failure, vision loss, metabolic syndrome, memory lapses, dementia

B. Causes include (but are not limited to)

- Age. The risk of high blood pressure increases as you age.

- Being overweight or obese. The more you weigh the more blood you need to supply oxygen and nutrients to your tissues. As the volume of blood circulated through your blood vessels increases, so does the pressure on your artery walls.

- Not being physically active. People who are inactive tend to have higher heart rates. The higher your heart rate, the harder your heart must work with each contraction and the stronger the force on your arteries. Lack of physical activity also increases the risk of being overweight.

- Using tobacco. Not only does smoking or chewing tobacco immediately raise your blood pressure temporarily, but the chemicals in tobacco can damage the lining of your artery walls. This can cause your arteries to narrow and increase your risk of heart disease. Secondhand smoke also can increase your heart disease risk.

- Too much salt (sodium) in your diet. Too much sodium in your diet can cause your body to retain fluid, which increases blood pressure.

- Too little potassium in your diet. Potassium helps balance the amount of sodium in your cells. If you don't get enough potassium in your diet or retain enough potassium, you may accumulate too much sodium in your blood.

- Drinking too much alcohol. Over time, heavy drinking can damage your heart. Having more than one drink a day for women and more than two drinks a day for men may affect your blood pressure. If you drink alcohol, do so in moderation. For healthy adults, that means up to one drink a day for women and two drinks a day for men. One drink equals 12 ounces of beer, 5 ounces of wine or 1.5 ounces of 80-proof liquor.

- Stress. High levels of stress can lead to a temporary increase in blood pressure. If you try to relax by eating more, using tobacco or drinking alcohol, you may only increase problems associated with high blood pressure.

C. Prevention

- Healthy diet

  i. Low salt

  ii.High potassium

- Healthy weight

- Physical activity

- No smoking

- Limiting alcohol

11. Obesity

A.Middle age is increasingly being linked to unhealthy weight gain due to more sedentary lifestyles

- Cardiovascular disease is the leading cause of death for men aged 35 and over.

B.Obesity is strongly linked to poor physical and mental health

12. Stress

    A. Common causes include but are not limited to

    - Having a heavy workload or too much responsibility
    - Working long hours
    - The death of a loved one
    - Loss of a job
    - Divorce
    - Increase in financial obligations

    B. Stress management tips (include but not limited to the following)

    - Positive attitude
    - Exercise regularly
        i. Your body can fight stress better when its fit
    - Eat healthy, well balanced meals
    - Rest
    - Prayer and meditation

13. Depression

A. One of the deadliest male health concerns for men over 40

- Up to 18% of the adult population
- Causes are similar to those of stress

B. Symptoms

- Become withdrawn
- Irritable
- Aggressive
- Hostile
- Lack of sexual desire
- Hide their feelings

C. Prevention

- Exercise
- Eat healthy (Foods that help fight depression)
    i. Vitamin D
    ii. Turkey/Chicken – Protein building-block tryptophan, which the body uses to make serotonin (plays a key role in depression)

iii.Brazil Nuts – Rich in selenium (People with less were more likely to get depressed)

   a.Brown rice, lean beef, sunflower seeds, seafood

iv.Carrots – Beta-carotene

   a.Pumpkin, spinach, sweet potatoes, and cantaloupe

v. Clams and Mussels – B-12

   a.Lack of B-12 causes a shortage of s-adenosylmethionine (SAM), which your brain needs to process other chemicals that affect your mood.

      • Lean beef, eggs

vi.Leafy Greens – Packed with folate (B-9)

   a.The brain needs folate to work well

      • Lentils, lima beans, and asparagus

vii. Salmon – High in polyunsaturated fats (omega-3 fatty acids) a.May help brain cells use chemicals that can affect your mood

- Also herring and tuna

- Sleep

- Skip alcohol

14. Liver Disease

A.Risk factors (include but not limited to)

- Heavy alcohol use

- Diabetes

- Obesity

B.Symptoms (include but not limited to)

- Super-itchy skin

- Eyes or skin turning yellow

- Gained a lot of weight suddenly

- Sudden weight loss

- Red palms

- Sleep schedule out of whack

- Memory has worsened

- Always tired

- Appetite disappeared
- Enlarged breasts (abnormal amounts of fatty tissue in the breast)
- Bruise easily
- Personality is changing
- Swollen legs and ankles
- Feel confused
- Body pains
- Feeling bloated
- Dark urine
- Can't concentrate
- Have the chills all the time
- Dry eyes and mouth
- Pale stool color, or bloody or tar-colored stool
- Nausea or vomiting

C. Prevention (include but not limited to)

- Drink alcohol in moderation
- Protect your skin

- Maintain a healthy weight

15. Diabetes

    A. One of the most common male health concerns over 40 even among men with low BMI's

    B. Type 2 diabetes is the most common form affecting men (90%-95%)

    C. Symptoms (include but not limited to)

        - Excessive thirst and hunger
        - Frequent urination (from uti or kidney problems)
        - Weight loss or gain
        - Fatigue
        - Irritability
        - Blurred vision
        - Slow-healing wounds
        - Nausea
        - Skin infections
        - Darkening of skin in areas of body creases

- Breath odor that is fruity, sweet, or and acetone odor
- Tingling or numbness in the hands or feet

D. Symptoms UNIQUE TO MEN

- Erectile dysfunction
- Retrograde ejaculation
- Low testosterone
- Decreased sex drive

E. Risk factors (include but not limited to)

- Family history
- Obesity
- Fat distribution: more fat around the middle
- High blood pressure
- High cholesterol
- Sedentary lifestyle
- Smoking
- Excess alcohol intake
- Lack of sleep low testosterone in men

- Unhealthy diet

F. Prevention and treatment (include but not limited to)

- Exercise regularly
- Control your carb intake
- Increase fiber intake
- Stay hydrated
- Implement portion control
- Choose food with a low glycemic index
- Control stress levels
- Monitor blood sugar levels
- Lose some weight
- Get quality sleep

16. Osteoporosis

A. After the age of 20 the body begins losing bone mass

B. Symptoms

- Backache
- Gradual loss of height and accompanying stooped posture

- Fractures of the spine, wrist or hip

C. Prevention

- Exercise

    i. Builds and maintains strong bones

- Calcium

- Vitamin D

- Magnesium, phosphorous, vitamin K, B, B12

- AVOID

    i. Diets rich in animal protein

        a. May cause calcium loss

    ii. Caffeine

        a. More than four cups of coffee per day inhibits calcium absorption and leads to calcium loss through the urine

    iii. Sodium

        a. Consuming too much salt causes loss of calcium through the kidneys

    iv. Smoking

        a. Makes it difficult for your body to use calcium

17. Colon Cancer

    A. One of the most common male health concerns over 40

- 1 in 22 risk of developing the disease in their lifetime, the bulk of them in men over 40

    B. Risk factors

- Being overweight or obese
- Physical inactivity
- Diets high in red meat and process meats
- Smoking
- Heavy alcohol use

    C. Prevention

- Staying at a healthy weight
  - i. Avoid weight gain around the midsection
- Physical activity
  - i. Vigorous activity has great benefits
- Limiting the red and processed meats and eating more vegetables and fruits lower your risk

- Avoid excess alcohol

- Not smoking

- Vitamins, calcium and magnesium Massage

KEITH'S FAVORITE EATS!

<u>Keith's Breakfast Tacos</u>

Ingredients:

- 2 whole eggs, 4 egg whites (from the shell)
- 4 coconut flour tortillas
- 4 whole cloves of garlic
- 1 cup of baby spinach
- 1 green onion
- 1/4 jalapeño pepper
- 4 tbsp of guacamole
- Canola oil spray or coconut oil spray
- 2 tsp each of crushed red pepper, oregano
- 1 tsp of black pepper

Directions:

1. Spray a small skillet with either of your choices of cooking oil and preheat on low heat.
2. Chop or combine baby spinach, garlic, jalapeño pepper, and green onion in a food processor and pulse to desired texture.
3. Add vegetable mixture to small skillet and cover. Let sauté for 4-5 minutes on low heat.
4. Spray a large skillet with your choice of cooking oil and preheat on medium heat.
5. Combine 2 large whole eggs and 4 egg whites in a mixing bowl with crushed red pepper, oregano and black pepper and mix well.
6. Pour egg mixture into large skillet, add vegetable mixture and scramble to your liking.
7. Remove egg and vegetable mixture and cover so it doesn't get cold.
8. Heat up the coconut flour tortillas directly on the gas stove fires on medium heat (my preferred method) or for 30-45 seconds in the microwave (depending on your microwave). This warms up the tortillas and improves the texture.

9.Place the tortillas on a large plate and spread 1 tbsp of guacamole on each.

10.Distribute the egg and vegetable mixture equally to each tortilla.

Nutrition Information:

Servings: 2

Per Serving: 267.5 calories, 10.7g total fat (3g sat. fat), 27g carbohydrates. (7.8g fiber), 17.2g protein, 437mg sodium

Keith's Famous Grilled Turkey Burger

Ingredients:

- 1/3 cup freshly chopped baby spinach
- 1 pound 99% lean ground turkey
- 3/4 tsp dried basil and oregano
- 1/4 tsp ground pepper
- 1/4 jalapeño pepper finely chopped

Directions:

1.Mix the turkey, baby spinach, basil, oregano, ground pepper and jalapeño in a large bowl. This will make 4 patties of equal size.
2.Lightly coat your grill (I use the George Foreman grill) with your choice of non-stick cooking spray (canola or coconut oil) and preheat.
3.Place the patties on the grill for about 4 minutes. The George Foreman type grills cook top and bottom at the same time so the amount of cook time may vary if you cook by a different means. Turkey this lean will easily overcook if you're not careful.

Top with your favorite burger dressings (lettuce, tomatoes etc.) These can be served with or without a bun. I like to use a gluten free bun and a tablespoon of guacamole.

Nutrition Information:

Servings: 1
Per Serving: 129 calories., 1.5g total fat (.5g sat. fat), 45mg cholesterol, 1g carbohydrates (.4g fiber), 26.6g protein, 111.4mg sodium

Healthy Salmon Dinner

Ingredients:

- 2 pounds of wild caught salmon (no dye)
- 5 springs of fresh rosemary
- 2-3 small lemons (sliced, with extra if desired)
- 2 tbsp extra virgin olive oil
- 1 tsp sea salt
- 1/4 tsp ground black pepper
- 4 cloves of fresh garlic (chopped)
- Smoked paprika
- Add fresh parsley or green onion if desired (chopped)

Directions:

1. Let salmon stand at room temperature for 10-15 minutes and preheat oven to 375 degrees F. Line a large baking sheet with foil.
2. Spray a thin coat of baking spray (I recommend canola oil spray) and place 2 springs of rosemary down the middle. Thinly slice one of the lemons and place half of the slices down the middle with the rosemary. Lay the salmon on top.
3. Evenly drizzle the salmon with the olive oil and sprinkle with the salt and pepper. Rub to evenly coat and add

the garlic over the top. Lay what's left of the lemon and rosemary on top of the salmon. Juice a second lemon and pour evenly over the salmon.

4. Fold the foil completely over the salmon, enclosing it. Leave just enough room for air to circulate inside. Cook 15-20 minutes until salmon is almost completely cooked through at its thickest point.

5. Take the salmon out of the oven and open the foil so the fish is completely exposed. Change the oven setting to broil and place the fish back into the oven and broil for a few minutes until the salmon and garlic are just a bit golden and the fish is cooked through. Be sure the salmon doesn't overcook and the garlic does not burn. As soon as the fish flakes with a fork, it's done.

6. Cut the salmon into desire portions and serve.

Nutrition Information:

   Servings: 6

   Per Serving: 180 calories, 6g total fat (1g sat. fat), 60 mg cholesterol, 4g carbohydrates (1g fiber), 28g protein

OVERCOMING OBSTACLES

People have a variety of reasons for not exercising. The most common excuse is simple boredom. People who aren't self-motivated to go to the gym don't view it as a fun or enjoyable place. To them it's just another place to work.

Time is another huge obstacle. What used to be a 9 to 5 job is more like a 7 to 7 job when you factor in the long commute. And once at home, the computer and cell phone have many still tethered to the workplace. Not to mention the fact that the spouse and children require time as well. If you have to travel out of town a lot for work, all of the above are compounded.

Last, but not least are injuries. They may be old injuries or simply a result of the wear and tear from getting older, but they limit movement. Of these nagging injuries, I hear about bad knees and back issues the most. It is very difficult to workout in pain especially in those areas, so I have listed some exercises that will make it easier for you to workout.

So, without further delay, lets overcome those obstacles to getting fit and being the best version of you!

MAKING EXERCISE FUN

1. Mix it up

   A.Go for a walk - you'll see things you haven't seen before - keeps it interesting

   - Take a different route

   - Take a hike

   - Spending time outdoors reduces stress, anger, depression, and brightens your mood

2. Bike riding

   A.Hit a trail

   B.Easier on the joints than running

   C.Stress reduction

   D.Fresh air

3. Listen to music, a podcast, the bible or motivational audio book during cardio

   A. Dance

   B. Keep your mind off of everyone else

   • Helps not to be concerned with who's watching

4. Bring a friend

   A. Motivate one another

   B. Fellowship

   C. Safer

   D. Continue exercising even if they don't show up

   • Strengthens your commitment and resolve

5. Accessorize

   A. Small weights or water bottles to challenge yourself

6. Compete – healthy competition

A. With friends

- "Myfitnesspal" and other apps allow you to connect with others in the fitness community

- "Exergaming" - video games that require physical participation

- "Meetup.com" for fitness groups

7. Set some reasonable goals

A. Hitting milestones keeps us excited about fitness

8. Relax

A. Chillin' out feels better when you've had a good workout.

B. You feel like you've earned it

9. Change up your workouts about every 6 weeks or so

A. Try some new exercises

B. Get in a class with others

C. Martial arts or self-defense classes

D. Pilates

E. Yoga

F. Dancing

• Zumba is a very popular and fun workout

10. Be your own cheerleader

A. Speak encouraging words over yourself and your training.

• You are strong

• You will reach your goals

• You will be consistent

• You will have fun sweating it out

B. Don't compare yourself to others, this is your journey

11. Set a reward – Something really desirable and maybe

a little frivolous

A. Buying a new outfit

B. Post-workout smoothie

C. Massage Journaling

12. Journaling

A. Keep a record of your journey and take pictures

• Looking at your progress is motivational

13. Avoid overtraining

A. Get your rest so you WANT to exercise again

B. Prevent injury

14. Turn your chores into exercise

A. You've got to do them anyway so why not make them fun and productive

• Change your mindset about the chores

- Carrying laundry up and down stairs

- Lifting groceries

- Scrubbing tubs and floors

- Gardening

- Spring cleaning

15. Hit the pool

A. Swimming is a challenging yet fun full body workout

B. Low impact

- Aerobic exercise that works all the major muscle groups without major impact to the skeletal system

- Every movement is a resistance exercise

C. Relaxing

QUICK WORKOUT FOR THOSE ON THE MOVE

This is a short workout that can be done at home or in a hotel room and with very minimal equipment or none at all. If you only have a few minutes to spare before you have to leave for that morning meeting this will be perfect for you. It is designed to get the maximum metabolic effect so no resting in between exercises unless absolutely necessary.

Notice that there is space to take notes on whatever you like. If you haven't worked out in a while I recommend taking notes on how your body feels during each exercise until you get accustomed exercising on a regular basis. Even if you feel great write it down.

Please, don't skip the warm up! Cutting corners can easily lead to injury and you can't workout if you're injured.

Terminology to know: A rep is how many times a movement is performed (repetitions). A set is a group of reps. So, you may perform 2 sets of 10 reps of lunges. This equals 20 reps.

WARM UP

EXERCISE	SETS	REPS	PHYSICAL NOTES
March or Jog in place	1	10	
Lunges with Twist	1	10	
Standing Knee Tucks	1	10	
High Kicks	1	10	
Push-ups	1	10	
Arm Swings/Rotations	2 (1 forward, 1 back)	10	

TRAVELERS WORKOUT

EXERCISE	SETS	REPS/TIME	PHYSICAL NOTES
Single Leg Lunge	1	8-10 each leg	
Squats or Squat Jumps with Side Arm Raises	1	8-10	
Push-ups	1	8-10	
Chair Dips	1	8-10	
Bird Dogs	1	8-10 each arm	
Planks	1	1 min.	
Side Plank	2	30 sec. each side	
Rest 30 Seconds and REPEAT			

EXERCISES FOR THOSE WITH KNEE PROBLEMS

1. Band Pull Throughs

A. Glutes

B. Hamstrings

2. Band Hip Rotations

A. Hips

B. Glutes

C. Quadriceps

3. Reverse Frog Hypers

A. Glutes

4. Wall Sit

A. Glutes

B. Quadriceps

5. Anterior Reach Lunge

A. Quadriceps

6. Straight Leg Deadlift

A. Glutes

B. Hamstrings

C. Lower back

7. Fire Hydrants

   A. Outer glutes

   B. Core

   C. Hips

8. Donkey Kicks

   A. Glutes

   B. Hip flexors

9. Clams

   A. Hip abductors

   B. Glutes

10. Monster Band Walks

   A. Glutes

   B. Hips

C. Quads

11. Side Shuffle

A. Glutes

B. Hips

C. Quads

12. Standing Band Abductions

A. Hip abductor

B. Glutes

13. Standing Band Kickbacks

A. Glutes

14. Seated Mini Band Abductions

A. Outer thigh

B. Glutes

15. Glute bridge with Mini Band

A. Glutes

B. Hip abductor

16. Glute Bridge and Curl

A. Glutes

B. Hip abductor

C. Hamstrings

D. Abs

17. Glute Bridge with Squeeze

A. Glutes

B. Hip abductor

C. Abs

18. Side Plank with Leg Raise

A. Obliques

B. Hip abductor

C. Glutes

19. Straight Leg Kick Back

A. Glutes

EXERCISES FOR THOSE WITH BACK PROBLEMS

1. Partial Crunches

B. Abs

2. Lying Hamstring Stretches

A. Lower back

B. Hamstrings

3. Wall Sits

A. Glutes

B. Quads

4. Press-up Back Extensions

   A. Stabilizing muscles in the back

5. Bird Dog

   A. Glutes

   B. Lower back

6. Knee to Chest

   A. Abs

7. Pelvic Tilt

   A. Glutes

   B. Lower back

8. Bridging

   A. Glutes

B. Hamstring

C. Abs/Core

9. Swimming

A. Full body with low impact

10. Clams

A. Hip abductors

B. Glutes

HIGH INTENSITY INTERVAL TRAINING FOR MEN 40 AND OVER!

This High Intensity Interval Training (HIIT) is designed to address the specific needs of men in their middle age years. It accomplishes this in a few different ways:

1. Burns a lot of calories in a short amount of time. In fact, it can burn up to 25-30% more calories than other forms of traditional exercises.

2. Speeds up the metabolism and keeps it higher for hours after exercise. HIIT has been found to shift the body's metabolism toward using fat for energy instead of carbs.

3. Helps you lose visceral fat. This is the disease-promoting fat surrounding your internal organs.

4. Promotes quality muscle growth (hypertrophy) especially in individuals who have not been active.

5. Improve oxygen consumption and increase endurance in a shorter amount of time.

6. Reduce blood pressure and heart rate.

7. Reduce blood sugar and improve insulin resistance.

In accomplishing the above, your body will be strengthened and enabled to combat a whole host of health concerns when performed in concert with proper nutrition.

I cannot stress enough how important it is for you to consult a physician prior to starting a training regimen. This may help you determine if you are healthy enough to begin an exercise program.

If any of the exercises cause you discomfort check to make sure you are performing the exercise correctly with good posture. The best way to do this is to look at your form in a mirror. If the discomfort remains, substitute an equivalent exercise.

There is space to log the weight you use as well as how you feel physically. I encourage you to utilize these sections. They will give you good information to use the next time you do those exercises.

I believe that it is highly important to warm up and stretch prior to and after each work out. Not only does it prevent injuries, but it promotes flexibility, reducing stress on the muscles and joints. Stretching makes the body feel really good!

Warm up

I recommend warming up on the elliptical machine if you have access to one. The elliptical has a low impact on our joints as opposed to a treadmill. It also has levers for your arms thus giving you the ability to warm up your lower and upper body effectively. This is important since this workout will essentially involve your entire body. If you don't have access to an elliptical machine or treadmill, the warm-up used for the Travelers Workout will do just fine.

Set the elliptical to the "Manual" setting and for 5 minutes.

For the first 3 minutes perform short, quick movements that mimic the actions of you quickly running up a flight of stairs 1 step at a time.

For the last 2 minutes perform long strides that mimic a sprint.

Stretching

When performing each stretch it is important to take your time especially if you have not stretched in a while. Be very deliberate and fluid with each motion. There is no reason to rush. If you're unsure of your form, look in a mirror. These are recommended stretches but there are so many more. If you desire to substitute other stretches feel free to do so.

| STRETCHES | | | |
EXERCISE	SETS	REPS	PHYSICAL NOTES
Alternating Back Lunge with Reach Up	1	5 ea. leg	
Alternate Toe Touches	1	5 ea. leg	
Lying Leg Cross Over	1	15 sec. ea. leg	
Page Turners	1	5 ea. arm	
Arm Swings	1	15	

Please note that these exercises are to be performed one right after the other with no rest (unless absolutely necessary) until it denotes REST.

DAY 1

Today's Motivational Scripture:

Proverbs 3:7-8 (NIV) *"Do not be wise in your own eyes: fear the Lord and shun evil. This will bring health to your body and nourishment to your bones."*

HIIT- DAY 1

EXERCISE	SETS	REPS/TIME	WEIGHT USED	PHYSICAL NOTES
Squats	1	8-12		
Leg Extensions	1	8-12		
Dumbbell Shoulder Raises (front and side)	1	8-10 front and side is 1 rep		
Jumping Jacks	1	45 sec.		
Hammer Curls	1	8-12		
Lunges	1	8-12		
Spider Planks	1	1 min.		

Congratulations, you finished your first day of HIIT! If you haven't worked out in a while or have never done this type of training you may be sore. That's okay. If you are overly sore you will want to adjust the amount of weight used prior to the next time you go through the Day 1 regimen. Use the "physical notes" and "weight used" columns to make note of the changes you need to make for yourself. This will help you customize your training. Additionally, take the next day off if necessary to rest. Otherwise, proceed with Day 2.

DAY 2

Today's Motivational Scripture:

Matthew 9:12 (NIV) *"On hearing this, Jesus said, It is not the healthy who need a doctor, but the sick."*

DAY 2			
EXERCISE	**SETS**	**REPS/TIME**	**PHYSICAL NOTES**
Elliptical Interval Setting	1	20 min.	
Alternating Back Lunge with Reach Up	1	5 ea. leg	
Alternate Toe Touches	1	5 ea. leg	
Lying Leg Cross Over	1	10 sec. ea. leg	
Page Turners	1	5 ea. arm	
Hurdle Stretch	1 each leg, hamstring and quads	10 sec. hamstring, 10 sec. quads	
Foam Roller	1	5-10 min. over body	

DAY 3

Today's Motivational Scripture:

Jeremiah 33:6 (NIV) *"Nevertheless, I will bring health and healing to it; I will heal my people and will let them enjoy abundant peace and security."*

HIIT- DAY 3				
EXERCISE	**SETS**	**REPS/TIME**	**WEIGHT USED**	**PHYSICAL NOTES**
Incline Bench Press	1	8-12		
Push ups	1	8-12		

Barbell Curls	1	8-12
Sumo Squats	1	8-12
Calf Raises	1	15-20
Crunching Jacks	1	10-15
Incline Dumbbell Flys	1	8-12
Burpees	1	8-12

Today's Motivational Scripture:

Proverbs 16:24 (NIV) *"Gracious words are a honeycomb, sweet to the soul and healing to the bones."*

DAY 4

You'll repeat the cardio and stretching from Day 2. Monitor your body, you may feel like you need a day of rest. If that's the case, take the day off to rest to get rejuvenated. Our muscles need time to repair and grow.

DAY 5

Today's Motivational Scripture:

1 Corinthians 9:24 (NIV) "Do you not know that in a race all the runners run, but only one gets the prize? Run in such a way as to get the prize."

HIIT- DAY 5

EXERCISE	SETS	REPS/TIME	WEIGHT USED	PHYSICAL NOTES
Cable Tricep Press	1	8-12		
Lat Pull Downs	1	8-12		
Dumbbell Deadlifts	1	8-12		
Leg Curls	1	8-12		
Jumping Jacks	1	45 sec.		
Seated Row	1	8-12		
Back Fly	1	8-12		
Butterfly Kicks	1	30 sec. to 1 min.		

DAY 6

Today's Motivational Scripture:

Isaiah 40:29 (NIV) "He gives strength to the weary and increases the power of the weak."

Day 6 is a fun day! I suggest getting outside for a leisurely walk for 30 minutes or so followed by some stretching. Take one of the suggestions from the list of things I provided to make exercise fun. Go for a relaxing swim or an easy bike ride. This will break up the monotony of being in the gym. Whatever you do on Day 6 should be VERY easy on the body because you have been through a tough week of training.

Week 1 Recap

Day 1: HIIT

Day 2: Cardio and Stretching

Day 3: HITT

Day 4: Cardio and Stretching

Day 5: HITT

Day 6: Day of Choice - Making Exercise Fun

After going through an entire week of HIIT it would be wise to go over your physical notes and the observations that you made about your body including how you felt. You will also want to review the amount of weight (if any) you were able to lift in conjunction with how you felt. Feel free to customize this workout to your liking. You may want to do more or less on specific days or take additional rest days. It's up to you.

Week 2

This week you will continue with the same schedule as Week 1 with a few tweaks to keep you both interested and challenged. Switch up what you did for fun on Day 6. Meditate on the same scriptures as Week 1.

Add a small amount of weight to the exercises (if you feel comfortable; "2.5-5 pounds is usually sufficient"). On the days you do HIIT, take 2 minutes of rest after the last exercise and repeat the routine a second time.

Substitute alternative exercises for those listed. For instance, substitute barbell curls for dumbbell curls, barbell squats for dumbbell squats, lunges for side steps, dips for tricep presses, flat bench press for dumbbell bench press, pull-ups for lat pull-downs, you get the point. There are a variety of substitutions (see my list below).

EXERCISE SUBSTITUTIONS

EXERCISE	BARBELL	DUMBBELL	MACHINE OR CABLE	BAND
Squats	Y	Y	Y	Y
Shoulder Raises (front and side)	Y	Y	Y	Y
Lunges	Y	Y	Y	
Bench Press	Y	Y	Y	
Curls	Y	Y	Y	Y
Sumo Squats		Y		Y
Calf Raises	Y	Y		
Pec Flys	Y	Y	Y	
Triceps Press	Y	Y	Y	
Lat Pull-Downs			Y	
Deadlifts	Y	Y	Y	
Row	Y	Y	Y	
Back Flys	Y	Y	Y	

Day 1: HIIT - Perform 2 sets of each. Add weight.

Day 2: Cardio and Stretching

Day 3: HITT - Perform 2 sets of each. Add weight.

Day 4: Cardio and Stretching

Day 5: HITT - Perform 2 sets or each. Add weight.

Day 6: Making Exercise Fun - Different activity

Week 3

This week you will continue with the same schedule as Week 1. Substitute exercises or keep the changes you made in Week 2. Check your notes, especially in the areas where you added weight. On Days 2 and 4, add 5 minutes to your cardio before stretching. On Days 3 and 5, add 1 set of side planks (1 min. each side) to the very end of your training. Switch up what you did for fun on Day 6. Meditate on the same scriptures as Week 1.

Substitute exercises and add a small amount of weight if desired to challenge yourself.

Day 1: HIIT - Perform 2 sets of each.

Day 2: Cardio and Stretching - 25 min. of cardio

Day 3: HITT - Perform 2 sets of each. Side planks.

Day 4: Cardio and Stretching - 25 min. of Cardio

Day 5: HITT - Perform 2 sets of each. Side planks.

Day 6: Making Exercise Fun - Different activity

Week 4

You have been committed to HIIT for 3 weeks! If you've been giving your body proper nutrition you definitely feel different than you did at the start of your training. Great job!

This week keep the weights the same on HIIT days as you lifted on Week 3. Strength comes in the form of control, speed, and endurance as well, not just in the amount of weight you can lift. After 3 weeks you have a good gauge on how much weight you can handle, so unless an exercise is simply not challenging, keep your weight the same. If you've been substituting exercises weekly, now would be a good time to go back and perform the exact same routine as in Week 1. Compare your notes afterward and see where you've progressed. Take your cardio up to 30 minutes on Days 2 and 4.

Day 1: HIIT - Perform 2 sets of each.

Day 2: Cardio and Stretching - 30 min. of cardio

Day 3: HITT - Perform 2 sets of each. Side planks.

Day 4: Cardio and Stretching - 30 min. of Cardio

Day 5: HITT - Perform 2 sets or each. Side planks.

Day 6: Making Exercise Fun - Different activity

Weeks 5-12 and Beyond

I encourage you to continue to make subtle changes to your training. The changes don't need to be major. They can be in the form of varied techniques that you've learned from research, the number of repetitions, more or less weight, or maybe bring a friend to work out with. Whatever you do, make it enjoyable and fun. Continue to meditate on the scriptures provided or add to them for your edification.

By the end of this 12-week journey, our desire for you is that there is life-altering change in your mind, body and spirit. Not only will you feel better, but you will BE better. By inviting God into every aspect of your life and further cultivating your relationship with the Father, you are on a healthy path to wholeness. I am truly honored to be a chosen part of your journey. I look forward to sharing in all of your success stories as you post them on our social media pages!

Keith's Prayer!

"Dear Heavenly Father, I thank You for the time, talent and treasure that You have so graciously and freely given to me that I might give it to others. Thank You Lord for the breath in our bodies, life, health and strength. I pray for a fresh anointing and a supernatural blessing for every participant of "Faithful, Forty & Fabulously Fit". Help them to keep their minds stayed on You as You lead them and guide them by Your most precious Holy Spirit through this 90 day training. Lord, I pray that as they build up strong vessels for Your use, that You also increase their self confidence. Teach them to hear Your voice even in the midst of training Lord and let Your Word be a lamp to their feet and a light to their path. At times they may feel like they are being tried in the fire, but let them come out even stronger and purified for Your glory. In the mighty name of Jesus, Amen!"

"Be a go-getter. And an ever better go-giver."

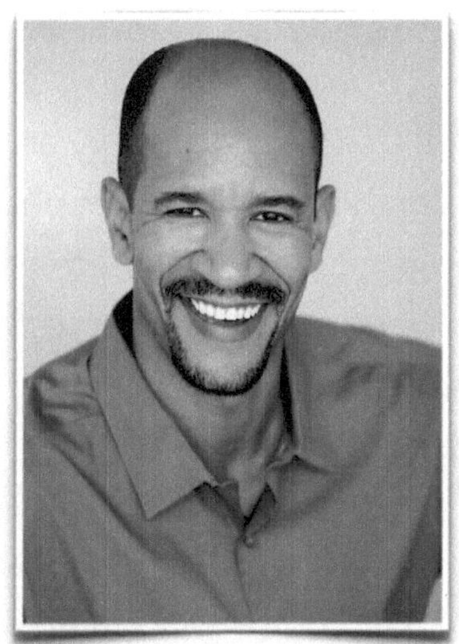

MEET
KEITH BOSSIER

Keith Bossier is a veteran Hollywood performer, screenwriter and award-winning physique competitor. Keith exudes passion and dedication. He takes great pride in having exceptional work ethic. His tireless study habits and extensive experience helped propel him into break out performances on the top-rated soap opera "The Young and the Restless" and multiple national commercials including "Capital One" and "Coke Zero". Some of his favorite works are his captivating performance as the co-pilot of flight 93 in "The Flight that Fought Back" and most recently, as an abusive father in the gritty drama, "The City".

As a creative, Keith wrote, starred in and produced VEL Productions maiden short film, "Potiphar's Wife". He is currently developing a feature-length, post-apocalyptic, action-adventure version of the same film. Keith has a vision to bring several Biblical stories to the big screen with a modern day flare.

When Keith isn't creating, he's engaged in jiu-jitsu, karate or in the gym. He is currently training with 7th degree blackbelt and Karate Hall of Famer, Sonny Garber. Personal growth is paramount to Keith, so in his off-time he enjoys learning Spanish, fitness modeling and motivating others to get fit for life. He's excited to add Spanish to his skill-set on his journey to being a positive, powerful and diverse force in Hollywood.

I enjoy sharing on social media! I can be followed on Instagram @phreed_fit, on Twitter @PHREED_fit and on Facebook @phreedfitness. Also, be encouraged to visit www.phreedfitness.com for upcoming events and exciting news!

ALSO BY ZONDRA WILSON

"RESTORATION! A JOURNEY OF FAITH IN OBTAINING
AND RESTORING GODLY RELATIONSHIPS!

"FAITH INTO ABUNDANCE: 30 STORIES OF FAITH
FROM SUCCESSFUL CHRISTIAN ENTREPRENEURS"

"MARRIAGE AND THE SINGLE LADY"

IF THIS BOOK HAS BEEN HELPFUL TO YOU, WE
WOULD LOVE TO HEAR YOUR PERSONAL STORIES OF
WHAT GOD HAS DONE IN YOUR LIFE.
SEND YOUR STORY TO:

zondraSwilson@yahoo.com
OR WRITE ZONDRA WILSON
12700 INGLEWOOD AVENUE
#1623
HAWTHORNE, CA 90251

JOIN OUR SOCIAL MEDIA SITES AT:
TWITTER - @FAITHFORTYFIT
FACEBOOK - @FAITHFULFORTYANDFIT
INSTAGRAM - @FAITHFULFORTYFIT